Milady's Standard Cosmetology Exam Review

Catherine M. Frangie

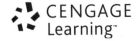

CENGAGE
Learning™

Australia • Brazil • Japan • Korea • Mexico • Singapore • Spain • United Kingdom • United States

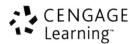
CENGAGE
Learning™

**Milady's Standard
Cosmetology Exam Review**
Catherine M. Frangie

For product information and technology assistance, contact us at **Cengage Learning Customer & Sales Support, 1-800-354-9706**

For permission to use material from this text or product, submit all requests online at **cengage.com/permissions** Further permissions questions can be emailed to **permissionrequest@cengage.com**

ISBN-13: 978-1-4180-4943-0

ISBN-10: 1-4180-4943-3

Milady
Executive Woods
5 Maxwell Drive
Clifton Park, NY 12065
USA

Cengage Learning is a leading provider of customized learning solutions with office locations around the globe, including Singapore, the United Kingdom, Australia, Mexico, Brazil, and Japan. Locate your local office at: **international.cengage.com/region**

Cengage Learning products are represented in Canada by Nelson-Education, Ltd.

For your lifelong learning solutions, visit **delmar.cengage.com**

Visit our corporate website at **www.cengage.com**

Notice to the Reader
Publisher does not warrant or guarantee any of the products described herein or perform any independent analysis in connection with any of the product information contained herein. Publisher does not assume, and expressly disclaims, any obligation to obtain and include information other than that provided to it by the manufacturer. The reader is expressly warned to consider and adopt all safety precautions that might be indicated by the activities described herein and to avoid all potential hazards. By following the instructions ?contained herein, the reader willingly assumes all risks in connection with such instructions. The publisher makes no representations or warranties of any kind, including but not limited to, the warranties of fitness for particular purpose or merchantability, nor are any such representations implied with respect to the material set forth herein, and the publisher takes no responsibility with respect to such material. The publisher shall not be liable for any special, consequential, or exemplary damages resulting, in whole or part, from the readers' use of, or reliance upon, this material.

Printed in the United States of America
7 11 10

Milady's Standard Cosmetology Exam Review

Foreword

This book of exam reviews contains questions similar to those that may be found on state licensing exams for cosmetology. It employs the multiple-choice type question, which has been widely adopted and approved by the majority of state licensing boards.

Groups of questions have been arranged under major subject areas. To get the maximum advantage when using this book, it is advisable that the review of subject matter take place shortly after its classroom presentation.

This review book reflects advances in cosmetology. It attempts to keep pace with, and insure a basic understanding of, sanitation, anatomy, physiology, and salon business applicable to the professional cosmetologist, client consultation guidelines, chemical safety in the salon, and basic procedures as well as some of the more advanced and creative aspects of the profession.

The book serves as an excellent guide for the student as well as for the experienced cosmetologist. It provides a reliable standard against which professionals can measure their knowledge, understanding, and abilities.

Furthermore, these reviews will help students and professionals alike to gain a more thorough understanding of the full scope of their work as they review practical performance skills and related theory. They will increase their ability to evaluate new products and procedures and to be better qualified professionals for dealing with the needs of their clients.

Part I: Exam Review for Cosmetology

CHAPTER 1—HISTORY AND CAREER OPPORTUNITIES

1. Which of the following civilizations was the first to infuse essential oils from the leaves, bark, and blossoms of plants for use as perfumes and for purification purposes?
   a. Chinese
   b. Egyptians
   c. Romans
   d. Greeks

   B

2. Archaeological studies reveal that haircutting and hairstyling were practiced in some form as early as:
   a. 1600 B.C. during the Shang Dynasty
   b. the Middle Ages
   c. 3000 B.C. in Egypt
   d. the Ice Age

   D

3. The art and science of beautifying and improving the skin, nails, and hair is:
   a. neurology
   b. cosmetology
   c. nail technology
   d. dermatology

   B

4. The first culture to cultivate beauty in an extravagant fashion was:
   a. the Greeks
   b. the Romans
   c. the Egyptians
   d. the Americans

   C

5. In 3000 B.C. the first recorded use of a hair-coloring agent was the use of:
   a. silver
   b. copper
   c. wax
   d. henna

   D

6. Hairdressing was an art during the time of the _____ for those who wore elaborate wigs and head dresses.
   a. Middle Ages
   b. Chinese
   c. Romans
   d. English

   A

7. During the Middle Ages, women wore colored makeup on their:
   a. ears
   b. hands
   c. lips
   d. eyes

   C

8. In ancient Rome, haircolor was used by women to indicate:
   a. personal wealth
   b. class in society
   c. marital status
   d. education level

   B

9. The barber pole has its roots of origin in what profession?
   a. medicine
   b. blacksmithing
   c. education
   d. psychology

   A

10. To achieve a look of greater intelligence during the Renaissance, women:
    a. wore highly colored lip preparations
    b. shaved their eyebrows and hairline
    c. wore elaborate, elegant clothing
    d. dyed their hair black or dark brown

    B

11. A popular method of adding color to the face during the Victorian Age was to:
    a. pinch the cheeks to induce natural color
    b. wear pale shades of rouge
    c. apply brightly colored preparations to the lips
    d. wear beauty masks made of natural ingredients

    A

12. In 1938, Arnold F. Willatt developed a method of permanent waving that used waving lotion with no heat called a:
    a. color wave   c. cold wave
    b. medium wave   d. hair wave

    C

13. In 1932, Charles Revson of Revlon marketed the first:
    a. nail polish   c. mascara
    b. commercial hair dye d. lipstick

    A

14. In 1998, Creative Nail Design introduced the first spa:
    a. payment system   c. pedicure system
    b. haircutting system d. color system

    C

15. To be a successful salon manager, it is important to have:
    a. styling skills   c. ability to manage people
    b. creative talent   d. inventory skills

    C

2

CHAPTER 2—LIFE SKILLS

1. Short-term goals can generally be completed in:
   a. one day
   b. one year
   c. one month
   d. one week

   B

2. A personal plan that will help you decide what you want out of life is called:
   a. goal mending
   b. compass setting
   c. goal setting
   d. harmony setting

   C

3. Long-term goals are measured in larger sections of time, usually:
   a. 5 to 10 years
   b. 5 to 10 months
   c. 7 to 12 months
   d. 5 to 7 minutes

   A

4. Making a list of tasks to complete from most to least important is called:
   a. personality
   b. penalty
   c. prioritizing
   d. personal

   C

5. The principles of good character are called:
   a. equal
   b. ethics
   c. embody
   d. enough

   B

6. Using discretion means:
   a. not sharing your personal problems with clients
   b. not repeating personal information clients have shared with you
   c. both a and b
   d. neither a nor b

   C

7. Being tactful means being straightforward but not:
   a. careful
   b. cautious
   c. critical
   d. clever

   C

8. A combination of understanding, empathy, and acceptance is called:
   a. sensitivity
   b. several
   c. secondary
   d. support

   A

9. That which propels you to do something is called:
   a. mutual respect
   b. visualization
   c. self-management
   d. motivation

   D

10. An unhealthy compulsion to do things perfectly is called:
    a. perfectionism
    b. performance
    c. personal
    d. priority

    A

CHAPTER 3—YOUR PROFESSIONAL IMAGE

1. When your personal appearance and conduct are in harmony with the beauty business, you project a:
   a. code of awareness
   b. work ethic
   c. personal glamour
   d. professional image

   D

2. One of the most vital aspects of good grooming is careful maintenance of:
   a. wardrobe
   b. finances
   c. exercise
   d. sensitivity

   A

3. The daily maintenance of cleanliness and healthfulness through certain sanitary practices is:
   a. personal creativity
   b. personal energy
   c. personal traits
   d. personal hygiene

   D

4. Your clothing should always be stylish and:
   a. functional
   b. formal
   c. highly accessorized
   d. colorful

   A

5. The inability to cope with a threat, real or imagined, is:
   a. relaxation
   b. personalities
   c. epidemic
   d. stress

   D

6. An important aspect of professional image is:
   a. physical attractiveness
   b. physical presentation
   c. physical problems
   d. physical activity

   B

7. The study of how a workplace can best be designed for comfort, safety, efficiency, and productivity is:
   a. ergonomics
   b. economy
   c. fatigue
   d. exposure

   A

8. The key to prevent repetitive motion injury is to be aware of:
   a. body posture and movements
   b. ill-fitting shoes and fatigue
   c. body manipulation and stress
   d. body vascular system

   A

9. Musculoskeletal disorders is a term used to describe:
   a. work-related repetitive injuries
   b. body-reducing fatigue
   c. extended periods of time
   d. varicose veins

   A

10. When providing client services, it is important to keep your back:
   a. elevated
   b. adjusted
   c. straight
   d. down

   C

CHAPTER 4—COMMUNICATING FOR SUCCESS

1. The ability to understand people is the key to:
   a. human relations
   b. operating inactively
   c. tension and misunderstanding
   d. operating effectively

   D

2. You are in a better position to do your job professionally when you:
   a. pay no attention to the motives and needs of others
   b. clearly understand the motives and needs of others
   c. pay some attention to the needs of others
   d. clearly ignore the motives and needs of coworkers

   B

3. Central to a stylist's success is:
   a. excellent customer service
   b. some customer service
   c. excellent coworkers
   d. ability to create conflict

   A

4. The single most important communication tool that should be done prior to any client service is the:
   a. body language
   b. release statement
   c. station preparation
   d. client consultation

   D

5. A form used to record information on a new client is also known as a:
   a. client questionnaire
   b. client appointment
   c. client request
   d. client recommendation

   A

6. Listening to a client and then repeating in your own words what you think the client is telling you is known as:
   a. valid suggestions
   b. reflective listening
   c. reflective thinking
   d. narrow selections

   B

7. To reiterate everything to a client during the consultation process means to
   a. repeat in measured, precise terms
   b. repeat in rapid, intense terms
   c. ignore the client's needs
   d. demonstrate the end results

   A

8. If you experience any problems with colleagues, the best way to resolve them is to:
   a. ignore them and do not speak to them
   b. speak with them directly and privately
   c. behave disrespectfully toward them
   d. speak to coworkers about them

   B

9. The individual in the salon that has the most responsibility for how the salon is run in terms of daily maintenance, operations, and client service is the:
   a. salon servicer
   b. salon manager
   c. salon client
   d. business partners

   B

10. Communication can be defined as:
    a. the art of effectively sharing information between two or more people
    b. the ability to solve problems and take quick action
    c. the art of ineffectively sharing information between two or more people
    d. the ability to trick the clients into having extra services

    A

11. An excellent time to discuss your progress with the salon owner or your employer is during a(n):
    a. coffee break
    b. lunch meeting
    c. employee evaluation
    d. client evaluation

    C

12. In the event that a situation is beyond your control, the key to handling your reactions is to:
    a. communicate past the issue
    b. argue with the client
    c. communicate that you are unhappy
    d. ignore the client's needs

    A

13. In handling a client who is dissatisfied with a service, the ultimate goal is to:
    a. argue with the client
    b. make the client happy
    c. make the client leave
    d. ask for specifics

    B

14. A good customer service practice to develop if you are behind schedule is to:
    a. have the client wait in the reception area until you are available
    b. call to inform your client about the delays
    c. have the client run other errands until you are available
    d. let the client wait and be inconvenienced

    B

15. To be successful, it is important for your career to:
    a. participate proactively by communicating your desires and interests
    b. be shy and not share your thoughts or questions with the salon manager
    c. be unprepared to discuss your desires and interests with the salon manager
    d. ignore positive feedback from the salon managers and coworkers

    A

CHAPTER 5—INFECTION CONTROL: PRINCIPLES AND PRACTICES

1. Material Safety Data Sheets (MSDSs) are obtained from:
   a. the EPA
   b. the salon manager or owner
   c. the product manufacturer
   d. OSHA

   ~~B~~ C

2. Regulatory agencies and governmental health departments require businesses that serve the public to:
   a. complete a self-evaluation procedure
   b. follow prescribed sanitary precautions
   c. create individual sanitary precautions
   d. have an employee orientation procedure

   B

3. Bacteria are very small and can only be seen with the aid of:
   a. a microscope
   b. a telescope
   c. bifocals
   d. a projector

   ~~C~~ A

4. One-celled microorganisms with both plant and animal characteristics are:
   a. boils
   b. bacteria
   c. decayed matter
   d. parasites

   B

5. In the human body, nonpathogenic bacteria help metabolize food, protect against infectious microorganisms, and:
   a. prevent gastrointestinal disorders
   b. stimulate the immune response
   c. stimulate the useful functions
   d. stimulate useful secretions

   D

6. Bacteria can exist:
   a. only on the skin or in the air
   b. only on porous surfaces
   c. only in water
   d. almost anywhere

   ~~B~~ D

7. A small minority of bacteria that cause disease when invading plant or animal tissue are:
   a. nonpathogenic
   b. phenols
   c. pathogenic
   d. antiseptics

   ~~B~~ C

8. A type of pathogenic bacteria that require living matter for growth are:
   a. phenols
   b. peroxide
   c. parasites
   d. viruses

   ~~B~~ C

9. Pus-forming bacteria arranged in curved lines that resemble a string of beads are:
   a. sterilization
   b. staphylococci
   c. superiority
   d. streptococci

   D

10. Cocci are pathogenic bacteria that are:
    a. round-shaped
    b. rod-shaped
    c. flat-shaped
    d. spore-shaped

    A

11. Bacteria that may cause strep throat or blood poisoning are:
    a. fungi
    b. spirilla
    c. bacilli
    d. streptococci

    D

12. Bacteria that grow in pairs and can cause pneumonia are:
    a. diplococci
    b. diphtheria
    c. discarded
    d. toxins

    A

13. Lyme disease, syphilis, or sexually transmitted diseases (STD) are caused by spiral or corkscrew-shaped bacteria called:
    a. flagella
    b. strep
    c. spirilla
    d. cocci

    C

14. In humans, pathogenic bacteria are known to produce:
    a. diseases
    b. disorders
    c. spores
    d. mitosis

    A

15. Bacteria that are transmitted through the air and rarely show active motility are:
    a. cocci
    b. bacilli
    c. epidemic
    d. disease

    A

16. Bacilli and spirilla bacteria are both motile and use slender, hairlike extensions known as:
    a. flat
    b. flagella
    c. spores
    d. spherical

    B

17. Harmless bacteria are what type of bacteria?
    a. nonpathogenic bacteria
    b. pathogenic bacteria
    c. general bacteria
    d. flagellum bacteria

    A

18. In 2000, a bacteria called *Mycobacterium fortuitum furunculosis* caused a client outbreak due to the failure of the practitioner to follow proper disinfection guidelines for:
    a. sharp implements
    b. whirlpool foot spas
    c. shampoo stations
    d. styling chairs

    B

19. Bacteria generally consist of an outer wall containing a liquid called:
    a. photographic
    b. photosynthesis
    c. protoplasm
    d. protons

    BC

20. The life cycle of bacteria has two distinct phases, the active stage and:
    a. inactive or spore-forming stage
    b. inactive and infectious stage
    c. inverted and growth stage
    d. inactive and revoked stage

    A

21. The process whereby bacteria grow, reproduce, and divide into two new cells is:
    a. mitosis
    b. membranes
    c. memory
    d. marriage

    A

22. Bacteria that pose little or no risk to a client in the salon setting but are dangerous in the medical setting are:
    a. daughter cells
    b. anthrax and tetanus bacilli
    c. tuberculosis and thorax
    d. acquired immunity

    B

23. The presence of pus is a sign of a(n):
    a. immunity
    b. nonpathogenic organism
    c. bacterial infection
    d. epidemic

    C

24. When body tissues are invaded by pathogenic bacteria, it is a sign of a(n):
    a. incision
    b. infection
    c. immunity
    d. spore

    B

25. Common human bacteria transferred through skin-to-skin contact or by using unclean implements are:
    a. saprophytes
    b. spores
    c. tetanus
    d. staphylococci

    D

26. When a disease spreads from one person to another, it is communicable or:
    a. contagious
    b. common
    c. corkscrew
    d. toxic

    A

27. An infection, indicated by a lesion containing pus, confined to a particular part of the body is a:
    a. frequent infection
    b. local infection
    c. primary infection
    d. poisonous infection

    B

28. When a disease spreads from one person to another by contact, it is:
    a. central
    b. disinfect
    c. contagious
    d. coughing

    C

29. A submicroscopic structure capable of infecting plants and animals including bacteria is a:
    a. motility
    b. mitosis
    c. virucide
    d. virus

    D

30. A virus can live and reproduce only by:
    a. improper use of sharp implements
    c. penetrating other cells and becoming part of them
    b. attaching to a bloodborne virus and becoming part of it
    d. poor personal hygiene

    C

31. Hepatitis A, a bloodborne virus, is marked by an inflammation of the:
    a. liver
    b. heart
    c. kidneys
    d. skin

    A

32. Human Immunodeficiency Virus (HIV) is the virus that causes:
    a. Intravenous Deficiency Syndrome
    b. Acquired Immune Deficiency Syndrome
    c. Acquired Immunity Syndrome
    d. Acquired Pathogenic Syndrome

    B

33. An organism that lives on another living organism and draws its nourishment from that organism is a:
    a. parasite
    b. pathogen
    c. favus
    d. contaminant

    A

34. If nail implements have not been disinfected properly, the client may contract:
    a. nail condition
    b. nail enhancements
    c. nail designs
    d. nail fungus

    D

35. Disease-causing bacteria or viruses that are carried through the body in the blood or body fluids are:
    a. bloodborne pathogens
    b. bloodborne capitis
    c. bloodborne elements
    d. bloodborne scabies

    A

36. Transmission of bloodborne pathogens can become possible through shaving, nipping, facial treatments, waxing, tweezing, or:
    a. sometimes if the skin barrier is broken
    b. anytime the skin barrier is broken
    c. when the skin is disinfected
    d. when the technician uses great care

    B

12

37. A skin disease caused by an infestation of head lice is:
   a. perpendicular   c. pediculosis
   b. scabies   d. peroxide

   C

38. The ability of the body to destroy pathogenic bacteria or viruses that have entered the body is:
   a. immunity   c. skin lesion
   b. epidemic   d. immigration

   A

39. The type of immunity the body develops after overcoming a disease or through vaccinations is:
   a. casual contact   c. acquired contact
   b. acquired immunity   d. an epidemic

   B

40. The surfaces of tools or objects not completely free from dirt, oils, and microbes are covered with:
   a. cholesterol   c. immunization
   b. containers   d. contaminants

   D

41. The process of removing pathogens and other substances from tools and surfaces is:
   a. decontamination   c. washing
   b. scrubbing   d. cleaning

   A

42. The three main types of decontamination are:
   a. disinfection, washing, and autoclave
   b. sanitation, disinfection, and sterilization
   c. sterilization, contaminants, and sanitation
   d. antiseptic, disinfection, and sterilization

   B

43. Decontamination is a process that involves the use of:
   a. physical and sensitive means to remove or destroy pathogens
   b. sanitation and the use of closed containers
   c. physical or chemical means to remove or destroy pathogens
   d. antiseptic practices and autoclaves

   C

44. Estheticians who use needles and probes that lance the skin must use a level of decontamination called:
   a. sterilization   c. phenols and bleach
   b. presterilization   d. dry heat sterilization

   A

45. In the salon setting, disinfection is extremely effective in controlling:
   a. microorganisms on non-living surfaces
   b. wet sanitizers on living surfaces
   c. soap and warm water
   d. disinfection procedures

   A

46. A higher level of decontamination than sanitation is:
    a. disinfection   c. discarded
    b. pathogenic   d. scrubbing   A

47. An exception to the level of protection that disinfection
    provides and the possibility of an infection could be present if:
    a. the client's skin is broken
    b. the client is washed and ready
    c. the item is given to the client
    d. the client has several services   A

48. A chemical agent that is used to destroy bacteria and viruses
    on surfaces is:
    a. 10% alcohol   c. antiseptic
    b. disinfectant   d. 20% peroxide   B

49. Disinfectants must have a registration number and be
    approved by the:
    a. Environmental Protection Agency (EPA)
    b. Occupation Protection Agency (OPA)
    c. U.S. Department of Labor (DOL)
    d. Food and Drug Administration (FDA)   A

50. A manufacturer must supply pertinent safety and storage
    information by providing:
    a. Material Storage Sheets   c. Material Safety Data
                                     Sheets
    b. Occupational Safety and   d. Material Forms and
       Health   Invoices   C

51. The agency that enforces safety and health standards in the
    workplace is:
    a. OSHA   c. DOL
    b. FDA   d. EPA   A

52. A disinfectant that meets regulatory agency requirements for
    destroying bacteria, fungi, and viruses is:
    a. bacterial, pathogenic, and virucidal
    b. bacterial, fungicidal, and virucidal
    c. bacterial, solvent, and disinfectional
    d. HIV, fungicidal, and sporicidal   B

53. A disinfectant used in salons should be appropriate and have
    the correct:
    a. efficiency   c. efficacy
    b. excellency   d. control measures   C

54. A salon implement that accidentally comes in contact with blood or body fluids should be cleaned and:
    a. completely immersed in an EPA-registered disinfectant
    b. washed and rinsed in an EPA-registered tuberculocidal antiseptic that kills HIV and HBV
    c. washed and placed in an EPA-registered antiseptic that kills HIV and hepatitis
    d. washed and immersed in an EPA-registered solution that kills HIV and AIDS

    A

55. Any item that cannot be disinfected after use on a client must be:
    a. washed   c. reused
    b. recycled   d. discarded

    D

56. Common, very safe, and useful types of disinfectant that contain sophisticated blends that work to disinfect implements in 10 to 15 minutes are:
    a. quaternary ammonium compounds
    b. quaternary peroxide antiseptics
    c. ammonium phenols and bleach
    d. 70% isopropyl alcohol

    A

57. Disinfectant with a high pH that can cause skin irritation or burn the skin or eyes are:
    a. alcohol and bleach   c. alcohol and quats
    b. EPA-registered   d. phenolic disinfectants
       disinfectants

    D

58. To be effective in the disinfection of implements, ethyl alcohol must be no less than:
    a. 20 percent   c. 75 percent
    b. 70 percent   d. 85 percent

    B

59. A common household product used effectively as a disinfectant is:
    a. sodium hypochlorite   c. formalin
    b. sodium alcohol   d. sodium hydroxide

    A

60. When mixing a disinfectant solution, add disinfectant to water and:
    a. mix more solution than is necessary
    b. mix equal parts of water and disinfectant solution
    c. mix according to the manufacturer's exact directions
    d. mix in sink areas to avoid spills

    C

61. To avoid contaminating implements, remove from a disinfectant solution using:
    a. tongs, basket, or gloves   c. bare fingers
    b. clean hands and fingers   d. middle finger and thumb

62. Store a clean, disinfected implement in:
    a. an open container at the station
    b. a station drawer with other implements
    c. an open drawer at the front desk
    d. a clean, dry container

63. How often must individual towels and linens be set aside to be laundered?
    a. after use on a client   c. at least once a week
    b. at the end of the day   d. no less than twice a month

64. The contact points of equipment that cannot be immersed in liquid solutions should be cleaned and disinfected using a:
    a. regulatory oversight agency approved disinfectant
    b. regulatory oversight agency approved antiseptic
    c. solution weaker than necessary
    d. solution that does not kill bacteria

65. At the end of the day, the disinfection procedure for a foot spa should include removing and cleaning the screen, washing the screen and inlet with soap and water, and totally immersing the screen in an approved disinfectant according to manufacturers' directions and:
    a. flushing with water and letting air-dry till the next day
    b. flushing the system with low-sudsing soap and warm water for 10 minutes, rinsing, draining, and letting air-dry
    c. removing the clean the screen if it appears dirty
    d. removing the screen and spraying it with a disinfectant solution

66. Every week, foot spas should be cleaned following the daily procedure and filled with:
    a. a disinfectant solution and left for 20 minutes, then drained and flushed
    b. a 10% bleach solution and left 10 minutes, then drained and flushed
    c. a disinfectant solution and left at least 6 to 10 hours, then drained and flushed
    d. a solution of hot soapy water

67. Any disposable material used in cleaning blood spills should be:
    a. placed in the recycle bin with the regular trash
    b. disposed of immediately
    c. placed in double bags before disposing or placed in a container for contaminated waste
    d. left at the station area

    C

68. The first step in the decontamination process is called:
    a. sanitation   c. antiseptic cleansing
    b. disinfection   d. surface wiping

    A

69. When using liquid soap, scrub your hands and lather for at least:
    a. 5 minutes   c. 1 minute
    b. 20 seconds   d. 10 seconds

    B

70. The use of bar soap is prohibited in most salons because bar soaps:
    a. are expensive   c. grow bacteria
    b. lather too much   d. lead to skin infections

    C

71. Which of these is a danger of using antibacterial soaps?
    a. They often do not kill germs and bacteria on the hands.
    b. They often cause the skin to dry quickly, causing fissures.
    c. They are ineffective in removing dirt and grime from the hands.
    d. They may promote the growth of resistant strains.

    D

72. Antiseptics are effective for:
    a. disinfecting instruments   c. disinfecting equipment
    b. sanitizing the hands   d. sterilizing equipment

    B

73. The agency that sets the standard for dealing with bloodborne pathogens is:
    a. OSHA   c. MSDS
    b. FBI   d. FDA

    A

74. Universal precautions require employees to assume that human blood and body fluids are infectious for:
    a. nonpathogenic pathogens   c. flu
    b. bloodborne pathogens   d. immunity

    B

75. A client that is infected with Hepatitis B or other bloodborne pathogens and shows no symptoms or signs of infection is:
    a. asymptomatic   c. healthy
    b. not infectious   d. in remission

    A

CHAPTER 6—GENERAL ANATOMY AND PHYSIOLOGY

1. Cosmetology is primarily restricted to the muscles, nerves, circulatory system, and:
   a. bones of the head, face, neck, arms, hands, lower legs, and feet
   b. bones of the legs, feet, and hands
   c. muscles and nerves of the head and face
   d. nerves and blood vessels of the hands, neck, face, and leg __A__

2. The basic unit of all living things is the:
   a. anatomy   c. muscle
   b. cell   d. nerve   __B__

3. The substance called protoplasm is found in:
   a. the cells of all living things   c. the structure of the human body
   b. the tissues and organs   d. inanimate objects   __A__

4. The study of the structures of the human body is:
   a. protoplasm   c. structure
   b. physiology   d. anatomy   __D__

5. A dense active protoplasm found in the center of the cell is:
   a. density   c. nucleus
   b. growth   d. structure   __C__

6. Most cells reproduce by dividing into two identical cells called:
   a. constructive metabolism   c. reproductive cells
   b. daughter cells   d. building cells   __B__

7. The watery fluid that cells need for growth, reproduction, and self-repair is found in the:
   a. cystine   c. cytoplasm
   b. anatomy   d. nerve tissue   __C__

8. The chemical process whereby cells are nourished and carry out their activities is:
   a. metabolism   c. membrane
   b. mitosis   d. memory cells   __A__

9. The chemical process of cell nourishment has two phases, which are:
   a. anabolism and catabolism   c. anabolism and repair
   b. reproduction and anabolism d. plasma and myology   __A__

10. A collection of similar cells that perform a specific function are:
    a. ligaments   c. tendons
    b. body fluids   d. tissue   __D__

11. A type of tissue that supports, protects, and binds together other tissues of the body is:
    a. nerve endings
    b. connective tissue
    c. coordinating tissue
    d. nerve tissue

    B

12. Tissues that are a protective covering on the skin or the lining of the heart and glands are examples of:
    a. epithelial tissue
    b. epidermis tissue
    c. exit tissue
    d. specific function tissue

    A

13. Nerve tissue is composed of special cells known as:
    a. respiratory tissue
    b. glands
    c. neurons
    d. tendons

    C

14. The physical foundation of the body is the:
    a. circulatory system
    b. muscular system
    c. integumentary system
    d. skeletal system

    D

15. The connection between two or more bones is a:
    a. tissue
    b. joint
    c. tendon
    d. muscle

    B

16. The scientific name for the study of the anatomy, structure, and function of the bones is:
    a. orthopaedic
    b. osteology
    c. trichology
    d. microbiology

    B

17. The ankle joint is formed by the tibia, fibula, and the:
    a. patella
    b. femur
    c. talus
    d. radius

    C

18. The oval, bony case that protects the brain is the:
    a. circle
    b. facial skeleton
    c. cranium
    d. occipital bone

    C

19. The hindmost bone of the skull, below the parietal bone, which forms the back of the skull above the nape is the:
    a. cranium bone
    b. occipital bone
    c. frontal bone
    d. temporal bones

    B

20. The bones of the face are involved in:
    a. facial expressions
    b. facial bridges
    c. facial massage
    d. connective tissue

    A

21. The system of the body that covers, shapes, and supports the skeleton tissue is the:
    a. muscular system
    b. muscular tissue
    c. respiratory system
    d. digestive system

    A

20

22. The medical term used to describe the study, function, and diseases of the muscles is:
    a. microbiology
    b. esthetics
    c. osteology
    d. myology

    D

23. The two bones that form the upper jaw are:
    a. nasal bones
    b. maxillae bones
    c. sternum bones
    d. cranium bones

    B

24. The two bones that form the sides and crown (top) of the cranium are the:
    a. parietal bones
    b. occipital bones
    c. nasal bones
    d. frontal bones

    A

25. The uppermost and largest bone of the arm, extending from the elbow to the shoulder, is the:
    a. carpus
    b. humerus
    c. phalanges
    d. radius

    B

26. The foot is made up of _____ bones.
    a. 16
    b. 26
    c. 18
    d. 24

    B

27. The _____ is a heavy, long bone that forms the leg above the knee.
    a. fibula
    b. ulna
    c. femur
    d. talus

    C

28. Muscles are fibrous tissue classified as three types, which are:
    a. buccinator, superior, and cardiac
    b. stretch, nonstretch, and cardiac
    c. cardiac, insertion, and striated
    d. striated, nonstriated, and cardiac

    D

29. Skeletal muscles attached to bone that are voluntary or controlled at will are:
    a. striated muscle
    b. cardiac muscle
    c. epicranius muscle
    d. trapezius muscle

    A

30. The part of the muscle that does not move is the:
    a. cardiac
    b. insertion
    c. origin
    d. tendon

    C

31. Pressure applied to a muscle during a massage is usually directed from the:
    a. middle to insertion
    b. beginning to end
    c. major to minor
    d. insertion to the origin

    D

32. The broad muscle that covers the top of the head is the:
    a. temporal
    b. epicranius
    c. deltoid
    d. occipital

    B

33. The front portion of the epicranius that raises the eyebrows, draws the scalp forward, and causes wrinkles across the forehead is the:
    a. frontalis
    b. occipitalis
    c. ligament
    d. temporalis

    A

34. The sternocleidomastoid muscle is the muscle of the neck that is responsible for:
    a. raising and lowering the eyes
    b. raising and lowering the arms
    c. lowering and rotating the head
    d. raising the mouth

    C

35. The ring muscle of the eye socket that enables the eyes to close is the:
    a. orbicularis minor
    b. posterior muscle
    c. orbicularis oculi
    d. serratus anterior

    C

36. A muscle covering the back of the neck and the upper and middle region of the back that rotates and controls the swinging of the arms is the:
    a. deltoid
    b. trapezius
    c. platysma
    d. zygomaticus

    B

37. Muscles that straighten the wrist, hand, and fingers to form a straight line are the:
    a. extensors
    b. digits
    c. deltoids
    d. biceps

    A

38. The muscles at the base of the fingers that draw fingers together are the:
    a. tendons
    b. abductors
    c. extensors
    d. adductors

    D

39. The gastrocnemius muscle is located in the:
    a. lower leg
    b. palm of hand
    c. mouth
    d. lower arm

    A

40. The scientific study of the structure, function, and pathology of the nervous system is:
    a. neutrons
    b. neurology
    c. myology
    d. osteology

    B

41. Every square inch of the body is supplied with fine fibers known as:
   a. neutrons
   b. platysma
   c. nerves
   d. cells

   _C_

42. The nervous system that controls the brain, spinal cord, spinal nerves, and cranial nerves is the:
   a. central nervous system
   b. voluntary nervous system
   c. peripheral nervous system
   d. spinal nervous system

   _A_

43. The system of nerves that carries impulses or messages to and from the central nervous system is the:
   a. involuntary nervous system
   b. respiratory nervous system
   c. mental nerve system
   d. peripheral nervous system

   _D_

44. The portion of the central nervous system that originates in the brain, extends down the lower extremity of the trunk, and is protected is the:
   a. spinal cord
   b. cell belly
   c. spinal atria
   d. nasal nerve

   _A_

45. The largest and most complex nerve tissue in the body is the:
   a. axon
   b. spine
   c. heart
   d. brain

   _D_

46. Whitish cords made up of bundles of nerve fibers held together by connective tissue are:
   a. neutrons
   b. nerves
   c. valves
   d. ventricles

   _B_

47. Sensory nerve endings that are located close to the surface of the skin are:
   a. receptors
   b. reactions
   c. capillaries
   d. spinal nerves

   _A_

48. Nerves that carry impulses from the brain to the muscles and produce movement are:
   a. median nerves
   b. motor cells
   c. spinal nerves
   d. motor nerves

   _D_

49. The largest of the cranial nerves, also known as the trifacial nerve or the trigeminal nerve, is the:
   a. fourth cranial nerve
   b. fifth cranial nerve
   c. supraorbital nerve
   d. maxillary nerve

   _B_

50. The chief motor nerve of the face that emerges near the lower part of the ear and extends to the muscles of the neck is the:
   a. digital cranial nerve
   b. efferent cranial nerve
   c. radial cranial nerve
   d. seventh cranial nerve

   _D_

51. The nerve and branches that supply the thumb side of the arm
    and back of the hand is the:
    a. buccal nerve   c. skeletal nerve
    b. radial nerve   d. posterior nerve   *B*

52. The anterior tibial nerve extends to the front of the leg, behind
    the muscles, and is also referred to as:
    a. dorsal nerve   c. saphenous nerve
    b. deep peroneal nerve   d. posterior auricular nerve   *B*

53. The system that controls the steady circulation of blood
    through the body by means of the heart and blood vessels is
    the:
    a. capillaries system   c. skeletal system
    b. circulatory system   d. lymph system   *B*

54. The system that involves the heart, arteries, capillaries, and
    veins is the:
    a. muscular system   c. digestive system
    b. blood vascular system   d. respiratory system   *B*

55. A clear yellowish fluid that circulates in the lymphatics of the
    body and carries waste and impurities away from the cells is:
    a. pericardium   c. lymph
    b. leukocytes   d. blood   *C*

56. The upper, thin-walled chambers of the heart are the:
    a. left and right pulses   c. left and right arteries
    b. left and right atria   d. left and right valves   *B*

57. The blood circulatory system that sends blood from the heart
    to the lungs to be purified is the:
    a. ventricle circulation   c. carotid system
    b. pulmonary circulation   d. lymphatic drainage system   *B*

58. Tubelike structures that include arteries, capillaries, and veins
    are:
    a. heart vessels   c. blood vessels
    b. valve vessels   d. platelet vessels   *C*

59. A thin-walled blood vessel that is less elastic than an artery
    is a:
    a. vein   c. leukocyte
    b. vulna   d. platelet   *A*

60. The largest artery in the human body is the:
    a. ventricle   c. aorta
    b. capillary   d. atrium   *C*

24

61. White blood cells perform the important function of destroying:
    a. nonpathogenic organisms
    b. disease-causing microorganisms
    c. internal and external movements
    d. carbon dioxide microorganisms

    B

62. The artery that supplies blood to the anterior (front) part of the scalp, ear, face, neck, and side of the head is the:
    a. lymph common artery   c. external carotid artery
    b. mandible cardiac artery   d. internal carotid artery

    C

63. The main blood supply of the arms and hands are the:
    a. facial and superficial arteries
    b. ulnar and radial arteries
    c. radial and posterior arteries
    d. ulnar and external jugular arteries

    B

64. Which of the following is NOT an artery that supplies blood to the lower leg or foot?
    a. popliteal artery   c. radial artery
    b. anterior tibial artery   d. posterior tibial artery

    C

65. Endocrine glands release a secretion called:
    a. platelets   c. enzymes
    b. hormones   d. perspiration

    B

66. The integumentary system is made up of the skin and accessory organs such as:
    a. oil and sweat glands, sensory receptors, hair, and nails
    b. diaphragm glands, secondary receptors, and nails
    c. involuntary glands, hair, and hands
    d. cardiac glands, voluntary glands, and nails

    A

CHAPTER 7—SKIN STRUCTURE AND GROWTH

1. The medical branch of science that deals with the study of skin, its functions, diseases, and treatment is:
   a. histology
   b. dermatology
   c. elasticity
   d. dermis

   B

2. The largest living organ of the body is the:
   a. lungs
   b. heart
   c. skin
   d. neck

   C

3. Healthy skin is slightly moist, soft, and flexible with a texture that is:
   a. soft and large pores
   b. smooth and fine-grained
   c. smooth and nonacidic
   d. rough and acidic

   B

4. Continued pressure on any part of the skin can cause it to thicken and develop a:
   a. callus
   b. infection
   c. rash
   d. psoriasis

   A

5. Appendages of the skin include hair, nails, and:
   a. oil and dirt glands
   b. sweat and keratin glands
   c. sweat and oil glands
   d. oil and pore glands

   C

6. The skin structure is generally thinnest on the:
   a. nose
   b. hands
   c. eyebrows
   d. eyelids

   D

7. The skin on the scalp has larger and deeper:
   a. nerve endings
   b. hair follicles
   c. keratin layers
   d. blood vessels

   B

8. The outermost layer of the skin is also called the:
   a. epidermis layer
   b. dermal layer
   c. thinnest layer
   d. second layer

   A

9. The epidermis layer of the skin does not contain:
   a. nerve endings
   b. sweat glands
   c. blood vessels
   d. sensory nerves

   C

10. The stratum germinativum is the deepest layer of the epidermis and is responsible for:
    a. growth of the epidermis
    b. strength of the epidermis
    c. nerve endings in the epidermis
    d. sweat and oil glands

    A

11. The dark special cells that protect sensitive cells and provide color to the skin are:
    a. reticular   c. dermis
    b. melanocytes   d. keratin   *B*

12. The granular layer of the skin is also called the:
    a. stratum granulosum layer   c. protective layer
    b. stratus melanocytes layer   d. adipose tissue layer   *A*

13. The outermost layer of the epidermis is the:
    a. fiber protein   c. lipids layer
    b. stratum corneum   d. second layer   *B*

14. A fiber protein that is the principal component of hair and nails is:
    a. keratin   c. sebum
    b. melanin   d. subcutis   *A*

15. The deepest layer of the epidermis is the:
    a. horny layer   c. stratum papillae
    b. stratum germinativum   d. clear layer   *B*

16. The clear, transparent layer under the skin surface is the:
    a. subcutaneous tissue   c. stratum lucidum
    b. stratum corneum   d. nerve cells   *C*

17. Cells that are almost dead and pushed to the surface to replace cells are shed from the:
    a. follicles   c. fatty skin layer
    b. stratum lucidum layer   d. stratum granulosum layer   *D*

18. The underlying or inner layer of the skin is the:
    a. dermis layer   c. keratin layer
    b. epidermis layer   d. basal layer   *A*

19. The outermost layer, directly beneath the epidermis, is the:
    a. clear layer   c. papillary layer
    b. dermal layer   d. elastin layer   *C*

20. The deepest layer of the dermis that supplies the skin with oxygen and nutrients and contains sweat and oil glands is the:
    a. regular layer   c. subcutis layer
    b. reticular layer   d. highly sensitive layer   *B*

21. Tissue that gives smoothness and contour to the body and provides a protective cushion is:
    a. subcutaneous tissue   c. epidermis
    b. sweat pores   d. basal cell layer   *A*

22. The clear fluid that removes toxins and cellular waste and has immune functions is:
    a. blood
    b. nerves
    c. corpuscles
    d. lymph

    D

23. Motor nerve fibers attached to the hair follicle that can cause goose bumps are the:
    a. arrector pili muscle
    b. body temperature
    c. sebum
    d. melanin

    A

24. Nerves that regulate the secretion of perspiration and sebum are:
    a. sweat pores
    b. melanocytes
    c. secretory nerve fibers
    d. tactile corpuscles

    C

25. Basic sensations such as touch, pain, heat, cold, and pressure are registered by:
    a. nerve fundus
    b. nerve endings
    c. light
    d. fear

    B

26. The amount and type of pigment produced by an individual is determined by:
    a. sun
    b. blood
    c. genes
    d. age

    C

27. Two types of melanin produced by the body are:
    a. brown and basal melanin
    b. keratin and elastin
    c. light and red melanin
    d. pheomelanin and eumelanin

    D

28. Skin gets its strength, form, and flexibility from flexible fibers found within the:
    a. dermis layer
    b. epidermis layer
    c. true skin
    d. scarf skin

    A

29. The fibrous protein that gives skin its form and strength is:
    a. granular
    b. melanin
    c. elastin
    d. collagen

    D

30. A fiber that gives skin its flexibility and elasticity is:
    a. elastin
    b. eumelanin
    c. melanin
    d. fibers

    A

31. The sudoriferous glands help the body regulate:
    a. dryness
    b. emotions
    c. temperature
    d. blood

    C

32. A tubelike duct that ends at the skin surface to form the sweat pore is the:
    a. arrector pili
    b. secretory coil
    c. follicle
    d. papilla

    B

33. The sebaceous or oil glands are connected to the:
    a. hair follicle
    b. adipose tissue
    c. nerve endings
    d. blood and lymph

    A

34. The principal functions of the skin are protection, sensation, heat regulation. excretion, and:
    a. flexibility and shape
    b. secretion and absorption
    c. strength and muscle tone
    d. hormone balance and repair

    B

35. The best way to support the health of the skin is by eating foods from:
    a. carbohydrates, vitamins, and water
    b. fats, oils, and vitamins
    c. water, dairy, and proteins
    d. fats, carbohydrates, and proteins

    D

CHAPTER 8—NAIL STRUCTURE AND GROWTH

1. The hard protective plate found at the ends of fingers and toes are:
   a. nail grooves
   b. natural nails
   c. nail ends
   d. mantles

   B

2. The area under a healthy nail plate should appear:
   a. bluish
   b. reddish
   c. pinkish
   d. brownish

   C

3. A main protein that is found in natural nails is:
   a. water
   b. keratin
   c. cuticle
   d. melanin

   B

4. Nails are an appendage of the skin and are part of what body system?
   a. digestive system
   b. respiratory system
   c. nervous system
   d. integumentary system

   D

5. A healthy nail is smooth, shiny, and:
   a. dark gray
   b. translucent gray
   c. bluish
   d. translucent

   D

6. The portion of the living skin on which the nail plate sits is the:
   a. nail bed
   b. cuticle
   c. nail fold
   d. ligament

   A

7. The nail bed is attached to the nail plate by a thin layer of tissue called the:
   a. natural nail
   b. free edge
   c. bed epithelium
   d. nail groove

   C

8. Nail cells are formed in what part of the nail structure?
   a. matrix
   b. mantle
   c. cuticle
   d. muscles

   A

9. The nail plate is guided and helped along during its growth by a thin layer of tissue called:
   a. matrix cells
   b. bed epithelium
   c. nail groove
   d. nail enhancement

   B

10. The matrix continues to create new cells provided that:
    a. it is conditioned with regular manicures
    b. it receives nutrition and is kept healthy
    c. it is attached to the free edge
    d. it extends beyond the free edge

    B

11. The visible part of the matrix that extends from underneath the living skin is the:
    a. cuticle
    c. lunula
    b. root
    d. bulb

    C

12. The most visible and functional part of the nail module is the:
    a. nail plate
    c. cuticle
    b. free edge
    d. lunula

    A

13. The nail plate is constructed of how many layers of nail cells?
    a. 10
    c. 50
    b. 20
    d. 100

    D

14. The part of the nail plate that extends over the tip of the finger or toe is the:
    a. free edge
    c. nail root
    b. manual edge
    d. nail groove

    A

15. The dead, colorless tissue attached to the nail plate is:
    a. groove
    c. cuticle
    b. matrix
    d. eponychium

    C

16. The living skin at the base of the nail plate covering the matrix area is the:
    a. eponychium
    c. cuticle
    b. hyponychium
    d. free edge

    A

17. The slightly thickened layer of skin that lies underneath the free edge of the nail plate is the:
    a. hyponychium
    c. eponychium
    b. cuticle
    d. nail fold

    A

18. Tough bands of fibrous tissues that connect bones are:
    a. arteries
    c. tendons
    b. ligaments
    d. mantle

    B

19. The slits or furrows on the sides of the nail plate are:
    a. artificial nails
    c. nail mantles
    b. natural nails
    d. nail grooves

    D

20. The length, width, and curvature of nails are determined by the:
    a. matrix shape
    c. groove shape
    b. bed epithelium
    d. furrow shape

    A

21. In the normal adult, the average rate of nail growth is about:
    a. 1/16 inch per month
    c. 1 inch per year
    b. 1/4 inch per month
    d. 1/10 inch per month

    D

22. A healthy natural nail will continue to grow provided there is no damage to the:
    a. cuticle
    b. groove
    c. matrix
    d. edge

    C

23. Replacement of the natural fingernail usually takes about:
    a. 6 to 12 months
    b. 4 to 6 months
    c. 4 to 8 weeks
    d. 2 to 8 months

    B

24. What fingernail grows the fastest?
    a. middle finger
    b. thumb
    c. toenails
    d. damaged nails

    A

25. The nail has a water content between:
    a. 10 and 15 percent
    b. 1 and 5 percent
    c. 20 and 45 percent
    d. 15 and 25 percent

    D

CHAPTER 9—PROPERTIES OF THE HAIR AND SCALP

1. The scientific study of hair, its diseases, and care is called:
   a. dermatology   c. biology
   b. trichology   d. cosmetology   *B*

2. The two parts of a mature hair strand are the hair shaft and:
   a. dermis   c. hair root
   b. hair follicle   d. hair ends   *C*

3. The portion of hair that projects above the skin is the:
   a. dermal papilla   c. hair root
   b. hair shaft   d. follicle   *B*

4. The follicle, bulb, papilla, arrector pili muscle, and sebaceous glands are main structures of the:
   a. hair shaft   c. cortex layers
   b. sudoriferous glands d. hair root   *D*

5. The tubelike depression or pocket in the skin or scalp that contains the hair root is the:
   a. follicle   c. bulb
   b. shaft   d. scalp   *A*

6. Hair follicles are not found on the palms of the hands or the:
   a. forehead area   c. soles of the feet
   b. elbow area   d. back of the neck   *C*

7. The follicle extends downward from the epidermis, where it surrounds the:
   a. epidermis layer   c. hair root
   b. dermal papilla   d. hair shaft   *B*

8. The lowest area or part of the hair strand is the:
   a. hair bulb   c. arrector pili
   b. hair shaft   d. sebaceous gland   *A*

9. A small, cone-shaped area at the base of the hair follicle that fits into the hair bulb is the:
   a. sweat pore   c. dermal papilla
   b. hair follicle   d. lymph gland   *C*

10. A tiny, involuntary muscle fiber inserted in the base of the hair follicle is the:
    a. dermal papilla   c. lanugo hair
    b. arrector pili   d. hair bulb   *B*

11. The oil glands of the skin connected to the hair follicles are:
    a. sweat glands
    b. dermal papilla
    c. sebaceous glands
    d. hair streams

    C

12. An oily substance secreted from the sebaceous glands is:
    a. sweat
    b. medulla
    c. sebum
    d. salt

    C

13. The overlapping layer of hair with transparent, scalelike cells is the:
    a. bulb
    b. follicle
    c. cuticle
    d. medulla

    C

14. The three main layers of the hair shaft are the cuticle, medulla, and:
    a. cortex
    b. shaft
    c. root
    d. bulb

    A

15. Swelling the hair raises the cuticle layer and allows for:
    a. primary defense
    b. penetration
    c. cross sections
    d. growth phase

    B

16. For chemicals to penetrate a healthy cuticle hair layer, they must:
    a. expose the mantle layer
    b. stiffen the hair shaft
    c. have an alkaline pH
    d. remove the cuticle layer

    C

17. The fibrous protein core of the hair, formed by elongated cells containing melanin pigment, is the:
    a. lower follicle
    b. cortex layer
    c. vellus hair
    d. dermal papilla

    B

18. The medulla is the innermost layer of the hair and is composed of:
    a. oval cells
    b. round cells
    c. coarse hair
    d. hair follicles

    B

19. Hair is composed of a protein that grows from cells originating within the:
    a. hair shaft
    b. hair follicle
    c. amino acids
    d. main elements

    B

20. The process whereby living cells mature and begin their journey up the hair shaft is:
    a. simplicity
    b. scalp
    c. keratinization
    d. medulla

    C

21. The five main elements that make up the chemical composition of human hair are carbon, oxygen, hydrogen, and:
    a. protein and amino
    b. cells and keratin
    c. elements and protein
    d. nitrogen and sulfur

    D

22. The chemical bonds that hold together the amino acid molecules are:
    a. convex bonds
    b. peptide bonds
    c. hydrogen drops
    d. protein cells

    B

23. An end bond is also known as a(n):
    a. molecule bond
    b. chain bond
    c. peptide bond
    d. elastic bond

    C

24. When peptide bonds hold together a very long chain of amino acids, it is called a:
    a. polypeptide chain
    b. hydrogen chain
    c. COHNS bond
    d. elasticity chain

    A

25. The three types of cross-links that form the bonds between the polypeptide chains are hydrogen bonds, salt bonds, and:
    a. disulfide bonds
    b. water bonds
    c. nitrogen bonds
    d. elastic bonds

    A

26. A weak type of physical side bond that is easily broken by water or heat is a(n):
    a. amino acid
    b. peptide chain
    c. single bond
    d. hydrogen bond

    D

27. A salt bond is easily broken with the use of:
    a. several acidic solutions
    b. conditioning treatments
    c. strong alkaline or acidic solutions
    d. thermal styling techniques

    C

28. Bonds that must be chemically separated are:
    a. disulfide bonds
    b. sulfur bonds
    c. cross links
    d. porosity

    A

29. Hydrogen chemical hair relaxers break disulfide bonds and during rinsing convert them to:
    a. COHNS bonds
    b. protein bonds
    c. sebum bonds
    d. lanthionine bonds

    D

30. The natural hair pigment found in the cortex layer of the hair is:
    a. melanin
    b. tissue
    c. protein
    d. brown

    A

31. Two different types of melanin are eumelanin and:
    a. phosphorus
    b. pheomelanin
    c. keratin
    d. sulfur

    B

32. Natural wave patterns are the result of:
    a. trichoptilosis
    b. health
    c. structure
    d. genetics

    D

33. Asians tend to have:
    a. extremely straight hair
    b. extremely curly hair
    c. straight to wavy hair
    d. wavy to curly hair

    A

34. Extremely curly hair grows:
    a. in long twisted spirals
    b. in short curves
    c. in a very regular pattern
    d. with very thick texture

    A

35. To help minimize tangles in extremely curly hair when washing, you should use:
    a. a drying shampoo
    b. strong scalp manipulations
    c. a detangling rinse
    d. regular soap instead of shampoo

    C

36. Extremely curly hair may often break or knot easily due to:
    a. humidity
    b. density
    c. high elasticity
    d. low elasticity

    D

37. Four important factors to consider in hair analysis are texture and porosity:
    a. elasticity and density
    b. dryness and length
    c. oiliness and length
    d. oiliness and color

    A

38. The thickness or diameter of the individual hair strand is the:
    a. hair strand
    b. hair porosity
    c. hair texture
    d. hair elasticity

    C

39. Hair texture is classified as:
    a. coarse, medium, or fine
    b. coarse, straight, or curly
    c. large or small diameter
    d. long, medium, or short

    A

40. The measurement of individual hair strands on one square inch of the scalp is:
    a. hair density
    b. hair structure
    c. hair length
    d. hair porosity

    A

41. The ability of the hair to absorb water or oil is:
    a. resistance
    b. porosity
    c. elasticity
    d. texture

    B

42. Chemical services performed on hair with low porosity require:
    a. neutral solutions
    b. more acidic solutions
    c. more alkaline solutions
    d. water solutions

    C

43. Hair with high porosity is often the result of:
    a. overprocessing
    b. conditioning
    c. too many shampoos
    d. hair texture

    A

44. The ability of the hair to stretch and return without breaking is:
    a. elasticity
    b. bounce
    c. porosity
    d. melanin

    A

45. Wet hair with normal elasticity will stretch up to:
    a. 25 percent
    b. 40 percent
    c. 50 percent
    d. 70 percent

    C

46. When shaping and styling hair, consider the hair's:
    a. length and color
    b. natural growth patterns
    c. natural shine and condition
    d. texture and color

    B

47. Dry hair and scalp can be caused by:
    a. inactive sebaceous glands
    b. alkaline water
    c. dry shampoos
    d. flaky scalp

    A

48. Oily scalp and hair can be treated by properly shampooing with:
    a. alkaline shampoo
    b. normalizing shampoo
    c. color shampoo
    d. warm water

    B

49. Hair that is not pigmented and almost never has a medulla is:
    a. oily
    b. pigmented
    c. dark
    d. vellus

    D

50. Long, soft hair found on the scalp, legs, arms, and bodies of males and females is:
    a. average
    b. scabies
    c. terminal
    d. vellum

    C

51. The phases of hair growth are anagen, catagen, and:
    a. telogen
    b. melanin
    c. repeated
    d. carbuncle

    A

52. The growth phase where new hair is produced is:
    a. transition
    b. telogen
    c. anagen
    d. regular

    C

53. The average growth of healthy scalp hair is:
    a. one half inch per week   c. three quarters of an inch
                                        per month
    b. one half inch per year   d. one inch per month   **D**

54. The final or resting phase in the hair growth cycle is:
    a. broken stage   c. anagen stage
    b. telogen stage   d. hypertrichosis stage   **B**

55. In general, the cross sections of curly hair can be:
    a. oval   c. even
    b. triangular   d. square   **A**

56. The term used to identify abnormal hair loss is:
    a. androgenic   c. areata
    b. alopecia   d. genetic   **B**

57. The sudden falling out of hair in round patches or baldness in
    spots is called:
    a. terminal hair   c. alopecia areata
    b. hypertrichosis   d. alopecia androgenic   **C**

58. Two products approved by the FDA to stimulate hair growth
    and allowed for sale in the United States are:
    a. minoxidil and finasteride   c. conditioning and rogaine
    b. tinea and medication   d. finasteride and antiseptics **A**

59. The technical term used to describe gray hair is:
    a. albinos   c. alopecia
    b. acquired   d. canities   **D**

60. A variety of canities, characterized by alternating bands of gray
    and pigmented hair, is:
    a. ringed hair   c. hypertrichosis
    b. alopecia areata   d. trichoptilosis   **A**

61. A condition of abnormal hair growth on areas of the body is:
    a. trichorrhexis   c. hypertrichosis
    b. hyperactive   d. electrolysis   **C**

62. Trichorrhexis nodosa is characterized by brittleness of the hair
    and the formation of:
    a. swellings along the hair shaft
    b. split ends along the hair shaft
    c. lubricated dry ends
    d. alternating bands of color   **A**

63. The technical term used to describe beaded hair is:
    a. monilethrix
    b. monoglycerine
    c. finasteride
    d. fragile

    A

64. The medical term for dandruff is:
    a. canities
    b. pityriasis
    c. alopecia
    d. simplex

    B

65. The medical term used to describe a fungal organism characterized by itching, scales, and painful circular lesions is:
    a. scapular
    b. seborrheic
    c. tinea
    d. alopecia

    C

66. The type of fungal infection characterized by red papules at the opening of the hair follicles is:
    a. tinea capitis
    b. pediculosis
    c. steatoides
    d. pityriasis

    A

67. A highly contagious skin disease caused by a mite parasite is:
    a. scabies
    b. capitis
    c. infestation
    d. furuncles

    A

68. An acute localized bacterial infection of the hair follicle that produces constant pain is:
    a. a furuncle
    b. scabies
    c. pediculosis
    d. carbuncle

    A

69. An inflammation of the subcutaneous tissue caused by staphylococci is:
    a. a carbuncle
    b. pediculosis
    c. anagen
    d. alopecia

    A

70. The spread of diseases can be prevented by practicing approved:
    a. healthy diet and exercise
    b. sanitation and disinfection procedures
    c. various options
    d. hair analysis procedures

    B

CHAPTER 10—BASICS OF CHEMISTRY

1. The science that deals with the composition, structures, and
    properties of matter and how matter changes under different
    conditions is known as:
    a. compounds   c. electricity
    b. chemistry   d. structural changes   **B**

2. The study of substances that contain carbon is referred to as:
    a. inorganic chemistry   c. organic chemistry
    b. chemical composition   d. natural products   **C**

3. Products manufactured from natural gas, oil, or plant or animal
    remains are considered to be:
    a. organic   c. inorganic
    b. natural   d. matter   **A**

4. Metals, minerals, water, and air are examples of :
    a. natural substances   c. compounds
    b. inorganic substances   d. proteins   **B**

5. Inorganic chemistry is the science that deals with compounds
    lacking:
    a. lead   c. carbon
    b. silver   d. water   **C**

6. Any substance that occupies space and has mass can be
    considered to be:
    a. simple   c. energy
    b. matter   d. inorganic   **b**

7. A basic substance that cannot be broken down into simpler
    substances without loss of identity is called:
    a. a compound   c. a molecule
    b. water   d. an element   **D**

8. Substances that cannot be divided into simpler substances by
    ordinary chemical means are:
    a. atoms   c. chemical
    b. inorganic   d. atomic   **A**

9. The smallest particle of an element is a(n):
    a. hydrogen   c. axle
    b. atom   d. acid   **B**

10. Chemically joining two or more atoms forms a(n):
    a. acid   c. mixture
    b. molecule   d. solvent   **B**

11. Chemical combinations of two or more atoms of different elements form:
   a. a mixture
   b. silicone
   c. oxygen
   d. a compound

   D

12. Normal matter exists in three different physical states, which are solid, gas, and:
   a. liquid
   b. organic
   c. air
   d. solute

   A

13. Characteristics that do not involve chemically changing a substance are:
   a. unique properties
   b. mechanical properties
   c. physical properties
   d. distinct characteristics

   C

14. A change in a substance's chemical composition is a:
   a. natural change
   b. chemical change
   c. chemical mixture
   d. chemical synthesis

   B

15. Matter that is not mixed with substances of different chemical compositions is a:
   a. pure substance
   b. physical substance
   c. chemical reaction
   d. compatible substance

   A

16. Physical mixtures containing two or more different substances are:
   a. suspensions, chemicals, and matter
   b. solutions, suspensions, and emulsions
   c. compounds, physical matter, and water
   d. minerals, compounds, and emulsions

   B

17. A blended mixture of two or more liquids or a solid dissolved in a liquid is a(n):
   a. solution
   b. emulsion
   c. compound
   d. alkaline

   A

18. A substance that dissolves another substance with no change in chemical composition is a:
   a. solute
   b. mineral
   c. solvent
   d. mixture

   C

19. Miscible liquids are liquids that can be:
   a. mixed without shaking
   b. mixed into stable solutions
   c. transformed into a suspension
   d. combined without a solvent

   B

20. Liquids that are not capable of being mixed into stable solutions are:
   - a. solutes
   - b. solvents
   - c. inverted
   - d. immiscible

   D

21. A product that does not separate when standing and contains particles is considered to be:
   - a. organic
   - b. a solvent
   - c. a solution
   - d. a mixture

   C

22. Solutions that contain undissolved particles that are visible to the naked eye are known as:
   - a. suspensions
   - b. mixtures
   - c. solutes
   - d. molecules

   A

23. A mixture of two or more immiscible substances united with the aid of a binder is known as a(n):
   - a. suspension
   - b. emulsion
   - c. mixture
   - d. solution

   B

24. A substance that acts as a bridge to allow oil and water to mix or emulsify is a(n):
   - a. active agent
   - b. surfactant
   - c. alkaline
   - d. deionization

   B

25. The water-loving head of a surfactant molecule is:
   - a. hydrogen
   - b. lipophilic
   - c. hydrophilic
   - d. neutral

   C

26. Ammonium hydroxide and ammonium thioglycolate are examples of products used to:
   - a. raise the pH of hair
   - b. neutralize the pH of hair
   - c. compose hydrogen bonds
   - d. neutralize the hair

   A

27. An atom or molecule that carries an electric charge is an:
   - a. arc
   - b. acid
   - c. ion
   - d. alkaline

   C

28. Acids owe their chemical reactivity to the:
   - a. chemical compounds
   - b. hydrogen ion
   - c. hydrogen peroxide
   - d. neutralization solute

   B

29. Chemical reactions that produce heat are called:
   - a. external
   - b. emulsions
   - c. redox
   - d. exothermic

   D

30. The chemical reaction that combines an element or compound with oxygen to produce an oxide is:
    a. suspension
    b. reduction
    c. neutralization
    d. oxidation

    D

31. The rapid oxidation of any substance accompanied by heat or light is:
    a. oxygen
    b. combustion
    c. protons
    d. electricity

    B

32. When oxygen is subtracted from a substance, the chemical reaction is called:
    a. release
    b. reduction
    c. oxidized
    d. redox

    B

33. A substance that has a pH above 7.0 is considered to be a(n):
    a. neutral solution
    b. acid solution
    c. alkali solution
    d. reducing solution

    C

34. A sweet, colorless, oily substance used as a moisturizing ingredient in cosmetic products is:
    a. glycerin
    b. moisturizing
    c. ointment
    d. compound

    A

35. The chemical reaction in which the oxidizing agent is reduced and the reducing agent is oxidized is:
    a. redox
    b. reducing
    c. neutral
    d. solute

    A

CHAPTER 11—BASICS OF ELECTRICITY

1. Electricity is described as a form of:
   a. energy
   b. movement
   c. negativity
   d. shortness
   ____

2. The flow of electricity along a conductor is called a(n):
   a. electric charge
   b. electric current
   c. swirl
   d. spark
   ____

3. Metals used in electric wiring and motors are materials that are considered good electricity:
   a. current
   b. conductors
   c. wattage
   d. ohms
   ____

4. Electric wires are usually covered with a rubber substance that is used as an insulator or:
   a. nonconductor
   b. mechanical
   c. current
   d. voltage
   ____

5. The path of electricity from the generating source through conductors and back to the original source is called a(n):
   a. electric charge
   b. alternating charge
   c. insulator
   d. complete circuit
   ____

6. Electric current that is constant, even-flowing and travels in one direction is:
   a. direct current
   b. direct volt
   c. converter
   d. active current
   ____

7. The device that changes direct current to alternating current is a(n):
   a. convex
   b. converter
   c. voltage
   d. ohm
   ____

8. A rapid and interrupted current that flows in one direction then in the opposite direction is:
   a. rectifier current
   b. alternating current
   c. active current
   d. direct current
   ____

9. The unit that measures the pressure or force that pushes the flow of electrons through a conductor is a(n):
   a. amp
   b. rectifier
   c. apparatus
   d. volt
   ____

10. The unit that measures the amount of electric current is a(n):
    a. battery
    b. volt
    c. ampere
    d. charger
    ____

11. The current that is used for facial and scalp treatments is
    measured in:
    a. milliamperes   c. wattage
    b. direct current   d. voltage   ____

12. The unit that measures how much electric energy is being
    used in one second is a(n):
    a. ohm   c. amp
    b. watt   d. volt   ____

13. The device that prevents excessive current from passing
    through a circuit is a(n):
    a. fuse   c. kilowatt
    b. battery   d. ampere   ____

14. A switch that automatically interrupts or shuts off an electric
    current at the first indication of an overload is a(n):
    a. voltage regulator   c. circuit breaker
    b. ampere current   d. battery charger   ____

15. An important way of promoting electrical safety is the principle
    of:
    a. grounding   c. low frequency
    b. connections   d. visible light   ____

16. An applicator that is used for directing the electric current from
    the machine to the client's skin is called a(n):
    a. steamer   c. polarity
    b. anaphoresis   d. electrode   ____

17. The positive electrode of an electrotherapy device is called
    a(n):
    a. frequency   c. vaporizer
    b. anode   d. accelerating   ____

18. The negative electrode of an electrotherapy device is called
    a(n):
    a. cathode   c. carbon
    b. electron   d. therapeutic   ____

19. The most commonly used modality that is a constant and
    direct current is:
    a. indirect current   c. galvanic current
    b. active current   d. Tesla current   ____

20. The process of introducing water-soluble products into the skin
    with the use of electric current is called:
    a. chemical reaction   c. iontophoresis
    b. inactive electrodes   d. electrodes   ____

21. A process that forces liquids into the tissues from the negative toward the positive pole is called:
   a. anaphoresis
   c. iontophoresis
   b. desincrustation
   d. therapeutic light
   _____

22. A thermal or heat-producing current with a high rate of oscillation that is used for scalp and facial treatments is:
   a. Tesla current
   c. alternating current
   b. direct current
   d. infrared current
   _____

23. Visible light, the part of the electromagnetic radiation spectrum that we can see, makes up what percentage of natural sunlight?
   a. 35 percent
   c. 60 percent
   b. 25 percent
   d. 50 percent
   _____

24. The long wavelengths that penetrate the deepest and produce the most heat are:
   a. infrared rays
   c. ultraviolet rays
   b. blue rays
   d. natural rays
   _____

25. To avoid damage to the eyes of a client or practitioner when using light therapy treatments, the eyes should be protected with saturated cotton pads or:
   a. safety goggles
   c. plastic cap
   b. sunscreen
   d. towels
   _____

CHAPTER 12—PRINCIPLES OF HAIR DESIGN

1. The foundation for all artistic applications is:
   a. space
   b. design
   c. design wave patterns
   d. design of parallel lines ____

2. The design process begins by analyzing the entire person and using the design elements and principles to:
   a. enhance positive features
   b. maximize negative features
   c. develop contrasting lines
   d. create transitional lines ____

3. In the hair design process, when deciding to take calculated risks, it is important to have a strong foundation in:
   a. confidence and balance
   b. fashion design
   c. techniques and skills
   d. form and space ____

4. In the principles of design, line defines:
   a. form and space
   b. less volume
   c. texture and form
   d. form and elements ____

5. Lines that extend in the same direction and maintain a constant distance apart are:
   a. design lines
   b. extended lines
   c. horizontal lines
   d. vertical lines ____

6. Lines positioned between horizontal and vertical, used to emphasize or minimize facial features, are:
   a. curved lines
   b. movement lines
   c. design lines
   d. diagonal lines ____

7. An example of a hairstyle created using a single line is a:
   a. contrasting style
   b. curved-line style
   c. monotone style
   d. one-length style ____

8. Curved lines that are used to blend and soften horizontal or vertical lines are:
   a. transitional lines
   b. styling lines
   c. contrasting lines
   d. parallel lines ____

9. The three-dimensional mass or general outline of a hairstyle is referred to as its:
   a. wave
   b. form
   c. weight
   d. line ____

10. In hairstyling, the area that surrounds the form is the:
    a. space
    b. line
    c. volume
    d. texture ____

11. Natural wave patterns are described as straight, wavy, curly, and:
    a. three-dimensional   c. combination
    b. very straight   d. extremely curly   ____

12. In hair design, with every movement, the relationship of form and what other design element change?
    a. space   c. texture
    b. volume   d. mass   ____

13. Hair texture changes can be created or changed temporarily with styling tools and permanently with:
    a. thermal styling   c. zigzag partings
    b. chemicals   d. flat irons   ____

14. Smooth wave patterns accent the face and can be used to narrow:
    a. a square jaw   c. a square chin
    b. rectangular features   d. a round head shape   ____

15. Illusions of dimension or depth are created when lighter and warmer colors are alternated with colors that are:
    a. darker and cooler   c. larger and darker
    b. smaller and closer   d. smaller and cooler   ____

16. For a client with gold skin tones, a flattering hair color tone would be:
    a. warm   c. contrasting
    b. cool   d. toned   ____

17. In the principles of art and design, the comparative relationship of one thing to another is called:
    a. space   c. proportion
    b. volume   d. harmony   ____

18. In designing for clients with large or broad shoulders, the stylist would create styles with:
    a. volume   c. classic
    b. length   d. shape   ____

19. Balance is described as creating equal or appropriate proportions to create:
    a. width   c. structure
    b. symmetry   d. space   ____

20. In designing, when the two sides are the same distance from the center, have the same length and volume, the balance is considered to be:
   a. symmetrical   c. asymmetrical
   b. even   d. similar   _____

21. In designing, when opposite sides have different lengths or different volume and appear to have equal visual weight, it is referred to as:
   a. rhythm balance   c. symmetrical balance
   b. positioned evenly   d. asymmetrical balance   _____

22. A recurrent pattern of movement in design is referred to as:
   a. rhythm   c. shapings
   b. diagonal   d. balance   _____

23. The area of a design where the eye is drawn to first before traveling to the rest of the design is called the:
   a. balance   c. emphasis
   b. axis   d. diagonal   _____

24. The most important art principle that holds a design together is:
   a. harmony   c. volume
   b. balance   d. emphasis   _____

25. The facial type that is about one and a half times longer than its width across the brow is the:
   a. oval face   c. facial contour
   b. oblong face   d. diamond face   _____

26. To offset or round out the features of a square facial shape, the aim would be to:
   a. create the illusion of width in the forehead
   b. add volume to top and closeness at the sides
   c. elongate the shape of the face
   d. create volume between the temples and jaw   _____

27. The facial shape with a narrow forehead and wide jaw and chin line is considered to be:
   a. square   c. triangular
   b. oval   d. diamond   _____

28. The face profile with a receding forehead and chin is generally referred to as:
   a. concave   c. straight
   b. circular   d. convex   _____

29. To give the illusion of proportional eyes to a client with wide-set eyes, the hair should be:
   a. slightly darker at the sides than top
   b. styled using a middle part
   c. straight lines at the jawbone
   d. full and below jaw   _____

30. The triangular section that begins at the apex or high point of the head and ends at the front corners is called the:
   a. crown area   c. line area
   b. bang area   d. convex area   _____

CHAPTER 13—SHAMPOOING, RINSING, AND CONDITIONING

1. The shampoo provides a good opportunity for the stylist to analyze the client's:
   a. hair and scalp conditions
   b. hair and facial features
   c. hair and makeup
   d. scalp and makeup
   _____

2. A client with an infectious disease should be referred to a:
   a. stylist
   b. treatment
   c. physician
   d. client
   _____

3. The primary purpose of a shampoo is to:
   a. recommend additional services
   b. cleanse the hair and scalp
   c. recommend products
   d. analyze scalp condition
   _____

4. In the shampoo selection process, understanding the pH scale helps the stylist:
   a. affect the look of a bad haircut for the client
   b. retail products to the client
   c. select the proper shampoo for the client
   d. determine an appropriate style for the client
   _____

5. An abundant and important element classified as a universal solvent is:
   a. salt
   b. soap
   c. detergent
   d. water
   _____

6. An alkaline shampoo with a high pH can leave the hair dry, brittle, and more porous and cause fading in:
   a. conditioning rinses
   b. color-treated hair
   c. relaxed hair
   d. virgin hair
   _____

7. Freshwater from lakes and streams is purified by the processes of sedimentation and:
   a. porous substance
   b. minerals
   c. filtration
   d. organic
   _____

8. Small amounts of chlorine can be added to water to:
   a. kill bacteria
   b. add minerals
   c. soften water
   d. add dimension
   _____

9. Water that contains certain minerals that lessen the ability of shampoo to lather readily is:
   a. rain water
   b. soft water
   c. hard water
   d. distilled water
   _____

10. In listing the ingredients of a product, the percentage of each ingredient is listed in:
    a. descending order   c. order of weight
    b. regular order   d. ascending order   _____

11. The second ingredient that most shampoos have in common is the primary surfactant or:
    a. color additive   c. conditioning agent
    b. preservative   d. base detergent   _____

12. The water-attracting end of a surfactant molecule is the:
    a. element   c. agent
    b. hydrophilic   d. hydroxide   _____

13. An acid-balanced shampoo has a pH in the range of:
    a. 4.0 to 6.0   c. 4.0 to 6.0
    b. 4.5 to 5.5   d. 5.0 to 5.5   _____

14. Shampoos that are recommended for use on color-treated or lightened hair are:
    a. alkaline-balanced   c. surfactant free
    b. detergent based   d. acid-balanced   _____

15. Shampoos with an acidic ingredient used to remove product buildup on hair are:
    a. clarifying shampoos   c. rinsing shampoos
    b. treatment shampoos   d. dandruff shampoos   _____

16. Shampoos used for oily hair and scalp that remove excess oiliness and keep the hair from drying out are:
    a. dry shampoos   c. balancing shampoos
    b. conditioning shampoos d. color-enhancing shampoos _____

17. Shampoos used to brighten or eliminate unwanted gold or brassiness are:
    a. color-enhancing shampoos c. neutralizing shampoos
    b. conditioning shampoos   d. conditioning shampoos _____

18. Substances that absorb moisture or promote the retention of moisture are:
    a. texturizers   c. shampoos
    b. melanins   d. humectants   _____

19. A product that slightly increases the diameter of the hair with a coating action, adding body to the hair, is:
    a. protein conditioner   c. color enhancer
    b. balancing treatment   d. instant conditioner   _____

20. A product that is used after a scalp treatment and before styling to remove oil accumulation is a:
    a. scalp neutralizer
    b. scalp astringent lotion
    c. balancing treatment
    d. conditioning treatment ____

21. Brushing of the hair should never be done prior to:
    a. chemical services
    b. shampoo services
    c. styling services
    d. conditioning services ____

22. The most highly recommended hairbrushes are those made from:
    a. nylon bristles
    b. thermal bristles
    c. natural bristles
    d. smooth bristles ____

23. To avoid physical problems during the shampoo, the correct posture is to:
    a. keep shoulders down and feet together
    b. stand as close as possible to the client
    c. keep shoulders back, abdomen in
    d. stand behind the client ____

24. After shampooing chemically treated hair, gently remove tangles beginning:
    a. at the front hairline and working down to the nape area
    b. at the nape and working up to the frontal area
    c. at the nape area and working sideways
    d. at the frontal area and work toward the ears ____

25. As a safety feature for the client, during a shampoo, the water temperature should be monitored by the stylist by:
    a. adjusting the volume and temperature of the water from hot to cold
    b. keeping one finger over the edge of the spray nozzle in contact with the water
    c. not adjusting the volume and the temperature of the water
    d. keeping the water pressure as high as possible for contact with one finger ____

26. Firm pressure and/or heavy scalp massage should not be administered during the shampoo procedure if the client is to receive a:
    a. client consultation
    b. leave-in conditioner
    c. conditioner pack
    d. chemical service ____

27. After a shampoo, it is not recommended to apply a conditioner:
    a. to the base of the hair, near the scalp
    b. midsection and ends of the hair shaft
    c. to the ends of hair shaft
    d. with massage movements ____

28. A shampoo that is performed when the client's health does not allow for a wet shampoo is a:
    a. dry shampoo procedure
    b. conditioning shampoo procedure
    c. weekly shampoo procedure
    d. medicated shampoo procedure
    _____

29. A stylist should recommend hair or scalp treatments only after performing a:
    a. scalp consultation
    b. professional service
    c. hair and scalp analysis
    d. shampoo procedure
    _____

30. A scalp treatment used when there is a deficiency of natural oil on the hair or scalp should contain:
    a. moisturizers and emollient ingredients
    b. sulfonated oil base products
    c. strong soap preparations
    d. mineral and greasy preparations
    _____

31. High-frequency current should never be used when the hair is treated with tonics that contain:
    a. dirt
    b. alcohol
    c. oils
    d. moisture
    _____

32. The overactive glands that produce excessive oiliness are the:
    a. hair follicles
    b. arrector pili glands
    c. sebaceous glands
    d. sweat glands
    _____

33. Dandruff is the result of a fungus called:
    a. malassezia
    b. scabies
    c. pathogenic
    d. tinea
    _____

34. Alcohol-based antidandruff lotions and tonics should not be used in conjunction with:
    a. thermal styling
    b. scalp massage
    c. filtration
    d. infrared lamps
    _____

35. When working a shampoo into a lather, the stylist should use:
    a. portion of nails
    b. cushions of fingertips
    c. long fingernails
    d. the wrists
    _____

CHAPTER 14—HAIRCUTTING

1. A good haircut begins with an understanding of the:
   a. body form
   b. head form
   c. body posture
   d. facial expression _____

2. The areas of the head where the surface of the head changes are:
   a. subsections
   b. starting points
   c. reference points
   d. apex points _____

3. In the haircutting procedure, reference points are used to establish:
   a. head shape
   b. design lines
   c. blunt cutting
   d. foundation lines _____

4. The widest part of the head, also known as the crest area, is the:
   a. apex area
   b. irregular area
   c. occipital area
   d. parietal ridge _____

5. The bone that protrudes at the base of the skull is the:
   a. occipital bone
   b. parietal bone
   c. frontal bone
   d. crest bone _____

6. The highest point at the top of the head is the:
   a. crown
   b. apex
   c. parietal
   d. occipital _____

7. The reference point that signals a change in head shape from flat to round or vice versa is the:
   a. crown area
   b. occipital corner
   c. four corners
   d. parietal ridge _____

8. The area at the back part of the neck below the occipital bone is the:
   a. guide area
   b. flat area
   c. ends area
   d. nape area _____

9. The triangle section that begins at the apex and ends at the front corners is the:
   a. fringe area
   b. front area
   c. corner area
   d. nape area _____

10. A thin continuous mark that is used throughout a haircut is called a(n):
    a. section
    b. corner
    c. angle
    d. line _____

11. The space between two lines or surfaces that intersect at a given point is a(n):
    a. corner
    b. angle
    c. bang
    d. line
    _____

12. The straight lines used to build weight or create a one-length or low-elevation haircut are:
    a. parallel lines
    b. horizontal lines
    c. weight lines
    d. diagonal lines
    _____

13. The straight lines used to remove weight or create graduated layers are:
    a. cutting lines
    b. diagonal lines
    c. vertical lines
    d. horizontal lines
    _____

14. The haircutting technique using diagonal lines to create fullness and blend long layers into short layers is:
    a. beveling
    b. weight
    c. diagonal
    d. fullness
    _____

15. For control during haircutting, the hair is divided into uniform working areas called:
    a. foundations
    b. uneven
    c. parts
    d. sections
    _____

16. The angle or degree at which a subsection of hair is held while cutting is:
    a. subsection
    b. elevation
    c. parting
    d. separating
    _____

17. Elevating the hair at 90 degrees or higher during a haircut results in the removal of:
    a. length and curl
    b. less graduation
    c. weight, or layering the hair
    d. bulk and length
    _____

18. The angle at which the fingers are held when performing a haircut is the:
    a. end shape
    b. blunt cut
    c. cutting line
    d. perimeter line
    _____

19. The first section cut when creating a shape is the:
    a. occipital line
    b. internal part
    c. guideline
    d. basic line
    _____

20. The outer line of a haircut is referred to as the:
    a. traveling guide
    b. stationary guide
    c. interior
    d. perimeter
    _____

21. The guideline used when creating layers or a graduated cut is a:
    a. traveling guideline
    b. outer guideline
    c. stationary guideline
    d. shape guideline _____

22. The technique of combing hair away from its natural falling position, rather than straight out from the head toward a guideline, is:
    a. subsectioning
    b. overdirection
    c. traveling guidelines
    d. undercutting _____

23. A conversation where the stylist offers professional advice and suggestions to the client is the:
    a. decision process
    b. suggestion process
    c. finished consultation
    d. client consultation _____

24. For a client with a long face, the stylist would recommend a style that:
    a. adds volume and height on top
    b. adds fullness on the sides to add width
    c. adds weight to chin and front
    d. adds fullness in length _____

25. To compensate for shrinkage associated with curly hair, the stylist should allow for shrinkage of:
    a. 1/4 inch to 1 inch
    b. 1/2 inch to 2 inches
    c. 1/8 inch to 1 inch
    d. 1 inch to 3 inches _____

26. The direction that hair grows from the scalp into a natural falling position is the:
    a. outermost perimeter
    b. growth pattern
    c. parallel section
    d. fringe area _____

27. The number of individual hair strands on one square inch of scalp is hair:
    a. texture
    b. crown
    c. density
    d. length _____

28. The haircutting tool with large teeth set far apart, designed to remove a significant amount of hair, is:
    a. haircutting shears
    b. edger shears
    c. clipper shears
    d. notching shears _____

29. A small haircutting tool used to create crisp outlines is a:
    a. feather blade
    b. trimmer
    c. razor
    d. texture shear _____

30. The haircutting tool used for close tapers in the scissors-over-comb technique is the:
    a. wide-toothed comb   c. tail comb
    b. barber comb   d. styling comb   ____

31. The hand that holds the shears, parts the hair, and cuts the hair during the cutting procedure is called the:
    a. holding hand   c. dominant hand
    b. right hand   d. extra hand   ____

32. The technique where the comb and shears are held closed in the dominant hand at the same time is called:
    a. palming the shears   c. opening the shears
    b. controlling the shears   d. holding the comb   ____

33. The technique used to free up the dominant cutting hand to cut a subsection is called:
    a. moving the shears   c. removing the shears
    b. transferring the comb   d. working the shears ____

34. A haircutting tool used for detailing and texturizing or an entire haircut is the:
    a. shingling   c. straight razor
    b. trimmer   d. carving   ____

35. The term used to describe the pressure applied to hair when combing or holding a subsection is:
    a. tension   c. elevation
    b. sectioning   d. angle   ____

36. When cutting straight hair to create a precise design line, use:
    a. no tension   c. tension ranges
    b. maximum tension   d. little tension   ____

37. When cutting hair, a general rule of thumb is to stand or sit:
    a. directly behind the area you are cutting
    b. directly in front of the area you are cutting
    c. indirectly behind the area you are cutting
    d. to the left of the area you are cutting   ____

38. In cutting uniform or increasing layers, the hand position most often used is cutting:
    a. at the fingertips   c. past the first knuckle
    b. between the fingers   d. over the fingers   ____

39. The technique of cutting below the fingers or inside the knuckles using a horizontal cutting line creates:
    a. cutting uniform or increasing layers
    b. heavier graduated haircut or a one-length bob
    c. shorter layer haircut or a shag effect
    d. high level layered effect or a bi-level cut

40. A haircutting technique that maintains control of a subsection with regard to elevations and overdirection is:
    a. cutting over the fingers
    b. cutting with a razor
    c. cutting palm-to-palm
    d. cutting below the fingers

41. When cutting below the finger, to prevent cutting the soft and fleshy part of the finger, avoid cutting past:
    a. the second knuckle
    b. the fingertip
    c. the index finger
    d. the thumb

42. The visual line in a haircut, where the ends of the hair hang together, is the:
    a. guideline
    b. weight line
    c. graduated line
    d. stationary line

43. A haircut achieved using a stationary guide and zero or no elevation and the hair comes to one hanging level is a:
    a. graduated cut
    b. long layers cut
    c. layer cut
    d. blunt cut

44. In a graduated haircut, the most common elevation used is:
    a. 0 degrees
    b. 45 degrees
    c. 80 degrees
    d. 30 degrees

45. Parting the haircut in the opposite way it was cut to check for precision of line and shape is:
    a. cross-checking
    b. consistent tension
    c. mirror elevation
    d. blunt cutting

46. The area of the head that has the most irregular growth patterns is the:
    a. nape
    b. back
    c. crown
    d. sides

47. In using the wide teeth of a comb when cutting, comb the section first with the fine teeth and then:
    a. change the position of the comb and comb with fine teeth
    b. switch comb to alternate hand and comb with fine teeth
    c. turn the comb around and comb with the wide teeth
    d. turn the comb on its side and comb with fine teeth

48. In general a razor should not be used on curly hair as it will:
    a. strengthen the weight line and cause the hair to frizz
    b. weaken the cuticle and cause the hair to frizz
    c. cause the hair to expand and the medulla to frizz
    d. strengthen the cuticle and cause the hair to flatten ____

49. The term used to describe how hair is moved over the head is:
    a. natural head form   c. natural fringe
    b. natural distribution   d. weight line ____

50. When working with a razor, the ends are cut at an angle producing a softer shape with more visible separation or:
    a. blunt effect   c. feathered effect
    b. short effect   d. geometric effect ____

51. A method of cutting or thinning hair where the fingers and shears glide along the edge of the hair to remove length is:
    a. angle cutting   c. slide cutting
    b. razor cutting   d. blunt cutting ____

52. The scissors-over-comb technique uses the comb to hold the hair in place and allows cutting from:
    a. side to side layers   c. alternating subsections
    b. extremely short to longer   d. slightly elevated sides
       lengths ____

53. The technique of removing excess bulk or cutting for effect without shortening hair length is:
    a. blunt cutting   c. texturizing
    b. angle cutting   d. compensating ____

54. Vertical point cutting performed with shears on the ends of hair:
    a. creates no effect   c. removes long hair
    b. removes gray hair   d. removes less hair ____

55. When performing the notching technique of texturizing with shears, the tips of the shears should be held:
    a. 5 inches from the ends   c. at the ends only
    b. 2 inches from the ends   d. at the midshaft section ____

56. Thinning hair to graduated lengths using a sliding movement with shear blades partially open is:
    a. slithering   c. point cutting
    b. notching   d. angle cutting ____

57. The slicing technique removes bulk and adds:
    a. stability through the lengths of the hair
    b. movement through the lengths of the hair
    c. layers and short lengths throughout the hair
    d. density through the lengths of the hair   _____

58. When performing the slicing technique on the surface of the haircut, it is best to work on:
    a. long hair   c. dry hair
    b. curly hair   d. wet hair   _____

59. A version of the slicing technique that creates a visual separation in the hair is:
    a. carving   c. thinning
    b. notching   d. pulling   _____

60. A tool attached to clippers that cuts the hair to the exact length is:
    a. clippers-over-comb   c. taper guard attachment
    b. length guard attachment   d. blended elevation   _____

61. With a regular cutting comb, the finer shaped teeth are geared for detailing, and the wider spaced teeth are geared for:
    a. slicing and angle cutting   c. combing and cutting
    b. removing length and detailing   d. edging a line   _____

62. When using the clipper-over-comb technique, the length is determined by the:
    a. apex of the head   c. size of the section
    b. angle of the comb   d. type of clipper used   _____

63. Cutting hair at the same length consistently, using a 90-degree elevation, produces a:
    a. uniform layer   c. one-length bob
    b. blunt cut   d. slide cut   _____

64. In the carving technique, to remove less hair, the scissors should be held:
    a. more open   c. more horizontal
    b. more closed   d. more vertical   _____

65. Clippers and trimmers should be cleaned and the detachable blade and heel disinfected:
    a. after each use   c. when needed
    b. daily   d. weekly   _____

CHAPTER 15—HAIRSTYLING

1. To ensure that the client has the knowledge necessary to care for their hair properly between salon visits, it is the responsibility of the professional to:
   a. never explain about proper home care maintenance
   b. educate clients on home hair maintenance and professional products
   c. suggest they purchase consumer products
   d. never suggest the use of professional products _____

2. The first step in the hairstyling process should always be a:
   a. cool water shampoo   c. client consultation
   b. draping procedure   d. conditioning treatment _____

3. Shaping and directing the hair into an S formation using a comb, lotion, and the fingers is called:
   a. hairstyling   c. ridge curls
   b. finger waving   d. roller setting _____

4. Hair gel that makes the hair pliable, keeps it in place, and is made from karaya gum is:
   a. conditioning gel   c. waving lotion
   b. diluted gel   d. hair conditioner _____

5. When creating finger waves with a side part, you should begin on the:
   a. drying side   c. control side
   b. heavy side   d. triangle side _____

6. In creating horizontal finger waves, the waves are placed:
   a. up and down the head
   b. on the heavy side of the head
   c. down and parallel
   d. sideways and parallel around the head _____

7. The stationary foundation of a pin curl is the:
   a. base   c. section
   b. curl   d. stem _____

8. The part of a pin curl that gives the curl its direction and movement is the:
   a. arc   c. base
   b. stem   d. no-stem _____

9. The stem of the pin curl is the part that determines:
   a. placement   c. width
   b. curl   d. mobility _____

10. Pin curls that produce tight, firm, long-lasting curls and allow for minimum mobility are:
    a. no-stem pin curl
    b. half-stem pin curl
    c. on-base pin curl
    d. off-base pin curl
    _____

11. Pin curls formed in a shaping should begin at the:
    a. open end
    b. closed side
    c. odd side
    d. shaping side
    _____

12. Smooth waves and uniform curls are produced by:
    a. closed center curls
    b. no-stem curls
    c. open center curls
    d. molded curls
    _____

13. Pin curls formed in the opposite direction of the hands of a clock are:
    a. alternating curls
    b. counterclockwise curls
    c. clockwise curls
    d. ridge curls
    _____

14. Pin curl bases are referred to as rectangular, triangular, square, or:
    a. arc-based
    b. on-base
    c. no-base
    d. closed-base
    _____

15. Triangular base pin curls are used along the front or facial hairline to:
    a. provide volume and height
    b. add wave patterns
    c. provide smooth overlapping curls
    d. prevent breaks or splits
    _____

16. Creating tension by forcing hair between the thumb and back of a comb when making pin curls is called:
    a. ribboning
    b. smoothing
    c. arcing
    d. placing
    _____

17. Pin curls sliced from a shaping and formed without lifting the hair from the head are:
    a. stem curls
    b. design curls
    c. carved curls
    d. ridge curls
    _____

18. Two rows of ridge curls placed on the side of a head are:
    a. ridge waves
    b. skip waves
    c. alternating waves
    d. clockwise waves
    _____

19. Pin curls that allow the hair to flow upward and downward are called stand-up curls or:
    a. cascade curls
    b. alternating curls
    c. C-shaped curls
    d. skip waves
    _____

20. Barrel curls are similar to a roller, but do not have the same:
    a. base
    b. tension
    c. volume
    d. angle _____

21. The panel of hair on which a roller is placed is the:
    a. stem
    b. section
    c. base
    d. subsection _____

22. Hair between the scalp and the first turn of a roller is the:
    a. curl
    b. base
    c. arc
    d. stem _____

23. For a roller set where little or no volume is required, the rollers should be placed:
    a. on-base
    b. off-base
    c. half-base
    d. down-base _____

24. The point where curls of opposite directions meet forming a recessed area is:
    a. indentation
    b. convex
    c. mobility
    d. directional _____

25. The metal edge of roller clips placed at an angle against the hair can cause:
    a. no tension
    b. long curls
    c. loose tension
    d. hair breakage _____

26. Combing small sections of hair from the ends toward the scalp creating a cushion or base is:
    a. back-combing
    b. combing sections
    c. comb-outs
    d. roller patterns _____

27. To smooth hair that is back-combed, the teeth of the comb or brush should be held at a:
    a. 15-degree angle
    b. 45-degree angle
    c. 90-degree angle
    d. 0-degree angle _____

28. When wrapping hair, very little volume will be attained provided the:
    a. style is correct
    b. hair at the scalp is not lifted
    c. hair is brushed smooth
    d. round brushes are used _____

29. The nozzle attachment used in blow-drying to create a steady stream of air is the:
    a. handle
    b. styling brush
    c. concentrator
    d. heating element _____

30. The tool attachment used to dry hair softly and accentuate the textural definition is a:
    a. diffuser
    b. nozzle
    c. concentrator
    d. texturizer _____

31. Teeth on a styling comb that are closely spaced remove curl definition and create a:
    a. textured surface
    b. shaped surface
    c. density surface
    d. smooth surface _____

32. Classic styling brushes having rows of round-tipped nylon bristles should be:
    a. heat sensitive and large
    b. heat resistant and antistatic
    c. heat resistant and narrow
    d. heat sensitive and heavy _____

33. An ideal brush for blow-drying fine hair quickly and adding lift to the scalp area is a:
    a. vent brush
    b. paddle brush
    c. grooming brush
    d. polish brush _____

34. A thickened liquid styling tool, spread with fingers, that creates the strongest control and distinct texture definition is:
    a. texturizer
    b. holding spray
    c. styling gel
    d. styling foam _____

35. A styling aid that holds fine hair with little or no heaviness is:
    a. heavy gel with weight
    b. holding spray
    c. texturizer
    d. pomade _____

36. A styling aid applied to damp wavy or curling hair to create a straight look when the hair is blow-dried is:
    a. styling foam
    b. straightening gel
    c. spray gel
    d. mousse _____

37. When blow-drying with a round brush, maximum lift is achieved by inserting the brush on base and directing the section up at a:
    a. slight angle
    b. back-and-forth motion
    c. 125-degree angle
    d. 45-degree angle _____

38. When using a concentrator to blow-dry straight or wavy hair, build the shape working from:
    a. left to right
    b. nape to crown
    c. top to bottom
    d. crown to sides _____

39. Waving and curling straight or pressed hair using special manipulative techniques on dry hair is:
    a. blow-drying
    b. thermal curling
    c. dry styling
    d. thermal rolling _____

70

40. The basic parts of a thermal iron are the rod handle, shell handle, and:
    a. barrel and shell
    b. heat regulator and stove
    c. bulb and barrel
    d. line handle and thermostat ____

41. The edge of a beveled flat iron that is nearest the stylist is the:
    a. inner edge
    b. control edge
    c. outer edge
    d. straight edge ____

42. To remove dirt, oils, and product residue from the barrel of a thermal iron, use a dampened towel with a soapy solution containing a few drops of:
    a. styling gel
    b. peroxide
    c. ammonia
    d. conditioner ____

43. Combs used with thermal irons should be about 7 inches long and made of:
    a. a flammable substance
    b. a plastic substance
    c. wide teeth
    d. a nonflammable substance ____

44. In thermal curling, hair is held at a 125-degree angle with medium tension and the curl is placed in the center if its base is a:
    a. full-base curl
    b. half-base curl
    c. thermal curl
    d. barrel curl ____

45. A type of thermal curl with only slight lift or volume can be achieved by using a 70-degree angle and:
    a. rolling hair completely off base
    b. rolling hair completely on base
    c. pushing the wave
    d. using liquid styling tools ____

46. A technique used to temporarily straighten extremely curly or unruly hair until the hair is shampooed is:
    a. hair pressing
    b. blow-drying
    c. thermal curling
    d. Velcro rollers ____

47. Applying a thermal pressing comb through the hair twice on each side to remove curl is a:
    a. hard press
    b. soft press
    c. thermal press
    d. medium press ____

48. Variations in hair texture are defined by the:
    a. length and style of the hair
    b. diameter and feel of the hair
    c. color and length of the hair
    d. color and style of the hair ____

49. Pressing wiry or curly hair requires more heat and pressure due to the:
    a. compact construction of the cuticle cells
    b. length and diameter of the cuticle cells
    c. diameter of the medulla cells
    d. texture and construction of the follicle cells ____

50. A tight scalp can be made more flexible with hair brushing and the systematic use of:
    a. conditioning masks   c. conditioning shampoos
    b. scalp massage   d. roller sets ____

51. The temperature of pressing combs should be tested:
    a. on a piece of light paper   c. on the client
    b. with running water   d. on a damp towel ____

52. To prevent the smoking or burning off of hair during the pressing treatment, avoid:
    a. excessive pressing oil   c. excessive tension
    b. excessive pressure   d. excessive pressing ____

53. When executing an updo, always inspect the shape you are building from every angle to determine:
    a. dimension and balance   c. length and building
    b. balance and proportion   d. texture and balance ____

54. A styling product available in a variety of strengths applied in the form of a mist to hold a style in position is:
    a. hair spray   c. foam
    b. mousse   d. liquid tools ____

55. A method of curling hair by winding a strand around a rod is a(n):
    a. pin curl   c. thermal curl
    b. on-base curl   d. spiral curl ____

CHAPTER 16—BRAIDING AND BRAID EXTENSIONS

1. In some African tribes, different styles of braiding signified a person's:
   a. personal bonds
   b. social status within the community
   c. fashion statement
   d. esthetic significance
   ____

2. Styling performed without chemicals or dyes and when the natural curl or coil pattern of hair is not altered is:
   a. traditional hairstyling
   b. natural hairstyling
   c. textured services
   d. unisex styling
   ____

3. To avoid misunderstandings in performing natural styling services, it is necessary to perform a(n):
   a. quality client consultation
   b. elaborate conditioning treatment
   c. excellent shampoo procedure
   d. preliminary scalp massage
   ____

4. When performing a consultation for natural hairstyling services, the focus should be on:
   a. service price
   b. time and effort
   c. hair length
   d. hair texture
   ____

5. In natural hairstyling services, texture refers to the diameter and feel of hair plus the:
   a. structure of hair
   b. condition of hair
   c. wave pattern
   d. length configuration
   ____

6. In textured hair, a coil configuration is defined as having a:
   a. square pattern
   b. tight curl pattern
   c. circular pattern
   d. loose curl pattern
   ____

7. To create length and soften facial lines with a square face, the hair should be styled with:
   a. waves and curls to create balance
   b. an updo style to create height
   c. a wave pattern to create depth
   d. a full style that frames the face
   ____

8. Styles with partial bangs or braids that frame the face and minimize a wide forehead should be used for facial shapes that are:
   a. round shaped
   b. an inverted triangle
   c. square shaped
   d. oval shaped
   ____

9. Hair with no previous coloring or lightening treatments, chemicals, or physical abuse is considered:
   a. chemical free hair
   b. textured hair
   c. structured hair
   d. natural or virgin
   _____

10. The brush recommended for scalp stimulation and removal of dirt and lint from locks is:
    a. vent brush
    b. boar-bristle brush
    c. nylon-bristle brush
    d. paddle brush
    _____

11. The bristles of a square paddle brush that are pneumatic will collapse when they encounter too much:
    a. resistance
    b. oil and dirt
    c. tension
    d. extension
    _____

12. The most important feature of a wide-toothed comb is the:
    a. distance between the teeth of the comb
    b. length of the comb handle
    c. colors available for the comb
    d. designs of the comb's teeth
    _____

13. A diffuser dries hair without disturbing the finished look or:
    a. dehydrating hair
    b. conditioning hair
    c. blending hair
    d. shortening hair
    _____

14. A manufactured synthetic fiber that does not reflect light and is similar in texture to extremely curly or coiled hair is:
    a. kanekalon
    b. yam
    c. nylon
    d. rayon
    _____

15. When curly hair is braided wet, it shrinks and recoils and may cause excess:
    a. matte finish
    b. slipping
    c. manufactured shine
    d. pulling and tension
    _____

16. To make straight or resistant hair more pliable when braiding, apply a:
    a. silicone shine spray
    b. light coat of wax or pomade
    c. heavy conditioner
    d. synthetic fiber
    _____

17. When blow-drying textured hair, the hair becomes soft and the wave pattern becomes:
    a. elongated
    b. sectioned
    c. combed
    d. tangled
    _____

74

18. The three-strand underhand braid technique where strands are woven under the center strand is a:
    a. twist braid   c. inverted braid
    b. visible braid   d. invisible braid   ____

19. The three-strand braid produced by overlapping the strands on top of each other is the:
    a. inverted braid   c. micro-braid
    b. box braid   d. visible braid   ____

20. The two-strand braid where the hair strands are twisted around each other is the:
    a. inverted braid   c. rope braid
    b. fishtail braid   d. visible braid   ____

21. In the fishtail braid, hair is picked up from the sides and added to the strands:
    a. as often as necessary
    b. as they are crossed over each other
    c. to make a third strand
    d. as they are split over each other   ____

22. Partings for braids can be square, triangular, or rectangular and determine:
    a. where the braid is placed and how it moves
    b. the length and direction of the finished braid
    c. the shape of the underhand or overhand technique
    d. the hair texture and where the braid is placed   ____

23. Extensions for single braids are integrated into natural hair using the:
    a. two-strand overhand technique
    b. three-strand underhand technique
    c. individual braid technique
    d. medium to large techniques   ____

24. Narrow, visible braids that lie close to the scalp created with a three-strand on-the-scalp braid technique are:
    a. french braids   c. fishtail braids
    b. cornrows   d. free-hanging braids   ____

25. Extensions added to cornrows or individual braids with the feed-in method build the braid up:
    a. with excessive weight   c. three stands as once
    b. using tension   d. strand by strand   ____

26. Natural textured hair intertwined and meshed together forming a single or separate network of hair is called:
    a. dreadlocks
    c. cornrows
    b. extensions
    d. braids _____

27. Three basic methods of hair locking are the comb technique, braids or extensions, and:
    a. networking
    c. block rolling
    b. meshing
    d. palm rolling _____

28. The gentle palm rolling method of locking hair takes advantage of the hair's natural:
    a. length and texture
    c. texture and diameter
    b. ability to grow
    d. ability to coil _____

29. The traditional cornrow is flat, natural, and:
    a. set in diagonal partings
    c. spiral in design
    b. contoured to the scalp
    d. overextended or misplaced _____

30. Synthetic hair fiber, human hair fiber, or yarn can be added to a single braid to form a:
    a. lock
    c. fishtail braid
    b. cornrow
    d. rope braid _____

CHAPTER 17—WIGS AND HAIR ENHANCEMENTS

1. The wig service costs and maintenance should be discussed during the:
   a. follow-up visit
   b. client consultation
   c. shampoo procedure
   d. fitting procedure ____

2. The artificial covering that covers 100 percent of the client's natural hair is a:
   a. toupee
   b. wig
   c. hairpiece
   d. braids ____

3. A small hair addition used to cover the top or crown of the head is a(n):
   a. braid
   b. extension
   c. hairpiece
   d. wig ____

4. The fastest way to determine whether a strand of hair is synthetic is to:
   a. burn it with a match
   b. ask the manufacturer
   c. shampoo the hair
   d. style the hair ____

5. With exposure, the color of human hair wigs may:
   a. last
   b. reset
   c. oxidize
   d. strengthen ____

6. Synthetic wigs that are particularly durable are made out of:
   a. silk
   b. polyester
   c. yak
   d. modacrylic ____

7. The most expensive wigs are constructed using:
   a. synthetic materials
   b. human hair
   c. monacrylic materials
   d. human hair mix ____

8. The root ends of hair with the cuticle placed in the same direction to prevent tangling is:
   a. human hair
   b. fallen hair
   c. tangle-free hair
   d. turned hair ____

9. A hand-knotted wig constructed for a secure fit with an elasticized mesh fiber base is a:
   a. connected weft
   b. cap wig
   c. capless wig
   d. synthetic wig ____

10. The hand-tied method of wig construction resembles actual hair growth with:
    a. flexibility at the root area
    b. availability in many colors
    c. ease of care
    d. special fitting requirements ____

11. A head-shaped form used for securing a wig is a:
   a. client
   c. block
   b. form
   d. canvas
   ____

12. When mounting a wig to a block, the wig should be pinned evenly using:
   a. bobby pins
   c. T-shaped pins
   b. staples
   d. H-shaped pins
   ____

13. When performing a haircutting procedure on a wig, the general goal is to make the wig:
   a. fit properly
   c. shorter
   b. achieve weight
   d. look realistic
   ____

14. When cutting a wig using a free-form method, move from longer to shorter lengths, working toward the:
   a. length
   c. sides
   b. weight
   d. form
   ____

15. Recommended styling products for wigs should be formulated for:
   a. color-treated hair
   c. textured hair
   b. natural hair
   d. synthetic hair
   ____

16. Before placing the wig on the head the hair should be:
   a. sectioned and secure
   c. wrapped and in rollers
   b. flat and even
   d. in pin curls and secure
   ____

17. When shampooing a wig, avoid shampoos that have a(n):
   a. oil base
   c. conditioning base
   b. sulfur base
   d. bolster base
   ____

18. Synthetic hair colors used on wigs and hairpieces are standardized using:
   a. natural color level ring
   c. 90 colors on the haircolor ring
   b. black to red color ring
   d. 70 colors on the haircolor ring
   ____

19. Prior to performing a color application on a wig or hairpiece, perform a:
   a. metallic test
   c. strand test
   b. patch test
   d. pulling test
   ____

20. Hairpieces with base openings that allow a client's hair to be pulled and blended are:
   a. full wig pieces
   c. interlocking hairpieces
   b. weft base hairpieces
   d. integration hairpieces
   ____

21. A small wig for men used to cover the top and crown of the head is a:
   a. toupee
   c. track
   b. wraparound
   d. weave   ____

22. Hair additions secured to the base of natural hair that add length, volume, texture, or color are:
   a. manufactured wigs
   c. hair wraps
   b. hair extensions
   d. hair combs   ____

23. Hair attached to an on-the-scalp braid that serves as the track is secured using a:
   a. track-and-sew method
   c. track-and-angle method
   b. glue-and-blunt method
   d. sew-and-diagonal method   ____

24. When sewing an extension onto a track, the needle should be:
   a. dull and pointed
   c. sharp and dull
   b. straight and long
   d. straight or curved   ____

25. The sewing stitch where the thread is wound around the needle twice is the:
   a. double-lock stitch
   c. overcast stitch
   b. secure lock stitch
   d. loop stitch   ____

26. Attaching hair wefts or single strands with an adhesive or glue is a:
   a. track method
   c. sewing method
   b. lockstitch method
   d. bonding method   ____

27. Hair that is bonded can be successfully shampooed provided it is done:
   a. gently
   c. weekly
   b. often
   d. monthly   ____

28. The fusion method of extensions requires that the bonding material be activated with:
   a. bonding materials and no pressure
   c. heat and finger pressure
   b. wefts and pressure
   d. heat from a special tool   ____

29. The fusion procedure involves wrapping both the client's hair and a:
   a. sectioned-based strip
   c. keratin-based strip
   b. free-form strip
   d. adhesive-based strip   ____

30. A styling maintenance program educates clients in the use of:
   a. styling products
   c. health issues
   b. client's budget
   d. catalog prices   ____

CHAPTER 18—CHEMICAL TEXTURE SERVICES

1. The chemical texture service that loosens overly curly hair into loose curls or waves is:
   a. curl softening
   b. curl re-formation
   c. alternate waving
   d. swelling compound ____

2. All chemical texture procedures involve changing the hair structure using:
   a. steady and constant changes
   b. chemical and layer changes
   c. physical and wave changes
   d. chemical and physical changes ____

3. The exterior hair structure layer that protects the hair from damage is the:
   a. cuticle
   b. medulla
   c. follicle
   d. shaft ____

4. The layer of the hair that provides strength and elasticity is the:
   a. medulla
   b. cortex
   c. regular
   d. arrector ____

5. Hair bonds that cannot be broken by heat or water are:
   a. disulfide bonds
   b. cuticle bonds
   c. sulfur bonds
   d. inner bonds ____

6. The natural pH of hair is between:
   a. 4.0 and 5.0
   b. 4.5 and 5.5
   c. 5.0 and 6.5
   d. 6.0 and 7.0 ____

7. One of the most important parts of a successful texture service is the:
   a. shampoo consultation
   b. client consultation
   c. draping procedure
   d. technical skill ____

8. Permanent waves cannot be performed if the hair is coated with:
   a. hydrogen shampoo
   b. metallic shine
   c. epsom salts
   d. metallic salts ____

9. Disulfide bonds are chemical-based side bonds that are formed when:
   a. three peptide bonds are broken apart
   b. sulfur atoms in two adjacent protein chains are joined together
   c. two salt-type chains are joined together
   d. three salt bonds are joined together ____

10. The measurement used to determine the hydrogen ions in a solution is:
    a. potential of hydrogen
    b. chemical composition
    c. potential negativity
    d. chemical solution ____

11. Chemical texturizers temporarily raise the pH of the hair by lifting the cuticle layer to:
    a. allow penetration to the medulla layer
    b. allow amino acids to swell
    c. allow penetration to the cortex layer
    d. allow keratin proteins to be removed ____

12. Long, coiled polypeptide chains that are part of the hairs structure are:
    a. salt bonds
    b. keratin proteins
    c. alkaline proteins
    d. peptide bonds ____

13. The client record card should include a complete evaluation of the length, texture, color, and:
    a. condition of the hair
    b. previous style of the hair
    c. client's favorite color
    d. the client's age ____

14. During the hair and scalp analysis procedure, the stylist should look for:
    a. cream conditioners
    b. abrasions or signs of scalp disease
    c. previous styling products used
    d. previous successful hair services ____

15. Hair texture that requires a longer processing or rewetting of solution to ensure complete saturation is:
    a. regular-textured hair
    b. fine-textured hair
    c. wavy-textured hair
    d. coarse-textured hair ____

16. The measurement of the number of hairs per square inch on the head is:
    a. density
    b. length
    c. porosity
    d. elasticity ____

17. An indication of the strength of the side bonds is:
    a. porosity
    b. elasticity
    c. flexibility
    d. absorption ____

18. The second process of a permanent wave is the:
    a. physical change process
    b. elasticity change process
    c. chemical change process
    d. influence change process ____

19. In permanent waving, the size of the curl is determined by the:
    a. position of the rod
    b. length of the hair
    c. wrapping of the rod
    d. size of the rod ____

20. The permanent wave rod that produces a uniform curl along the entire width of the strand is a:
    a. straight rod
    b. concave rod
    c. convex rod
    d. loop rod ____

21. A wrapping technique using two endpapers, one placed under the strand and one over is the:
    a. bookend wrap
    b. double-flat wrap
    c. single-flat wrap
    d. end wrap ____

22. Permanent wave rods are placed onto subsections of a panel called:
    a. base sections
    b. panel sections
    c. inverted sections
    d. center sections ____

23. The position of a permanent wave rod in relation to its base section is the:
    a. base direction
    b. rod angle
    c. wrapping angle
    d. base placement ____

24. The technique of wrapping at a 90-degree angle or straight out from the center is:
    a. half-off base placement
    b. base direction placement
    c. greater volume placement
    d. lesser volume placement ____

25. The two basic types of wrapping hair around a perm rod are the spiral method and:
    a. loop method
    b. croquignole method
    c. placement method
    d. horizontal method ____

26. A technique used to wrap extra-long hair using two rods in opposite directions is a(n):
    a. croquignole perm wrap
    b. ends perm wrap
    c. piggyback wrap
    d. spiral perm wrap ____

27. A reduction reaction involves either the addition of hydrogen or removal of:
    a. oxygen
    b. peroxide
    c. carbon
    d. nitrogen ____

28. A common, colorless reducing agent used in chemical texture services is:
    a. alkalizing agent
    b. thioglycolic acid
    c. reducing agent
    d. endothermic acid ____

29. The main reducing agent in alkaline permanents is:
    a. sodium hydroxide
    b. ammonium thioglycolate
    c. ammonium hydroxide
    d. ammonium bromide _____

30. Most alkaline permanent waves have a pH between:
    a. 9.0 and 9.6
    b. 9.0 and 10.1
    c. 8.0 and 10.0
    d. 9.5 and 10.1 _____

31. The primary low pH reducing agent in acid waves is:
    a. ammonium hydroxide
    b. glyceryl monothermic
    c. ammonium thioglycolate
    d. glyceryl monothioglycolate _____

32. An exothermic chemical reaction produces:
    a. thio
    b. heat
    c. hydrogen
    d. reactions _____

33. The basic components of acid waves are permanent wave solution and:
    a. conditioner and activator
    b. neutralizer and stabilizer
    c. activator and neutralizer
    d. shampoo and neutralizer _____

34. An endothermic wave must be activated using a(n):
    a. ammonia lotion
    b. outside heat source
    c. sulfite source
    d. reducing agent _____

35. In permanent waving, the processing should be determined by the:
    a. strength of the solution
    b. size of the rods
    c. processing time
    d. length of the hair _____

36. Hair that is too weak to hold a curl or may be completely straight after a perm is:
    a. overcurly
    b. over-processed
    c. oversaturated
    d. underprocessed _____

37. The process of stopping the action of a permanent wave is:
    a. rinsing
    b. rebuilding
    c. normalizing
    d. neutralization _____

38. Permanent wave solution should be rinsed from the hair for a minimum of:
    a. 2 minutes
    b. 10 minutes
    c. 5 minutes
    d. 15 minutes _____

39. A 90-degree perm wrap that minimizes stress and tension on the hair is:
    a. half off base
    b. on base
    c. overdirected
    d. curved base _____

40. The process of rearranging extremely curly hair into a straighter or smoother form is:
    a. chemical hair relaxing
    b. chemical smoothing
    c. continuation
    d. neutralizing
    _____

41. In extremely curly hair, the thinnest and weakest sections of the hair strand are located at the:
    a. twists
    b. roots
    c. diameter
    d. shaft
    _____

42. Thio chemical relaxers usually have a pH value above:
    a. 5
    b. 10
    c. 9
    d. 6
    _____

43. The active ingredient in all hydroxide relaxers is the hydroxide:
    a. viscosity
    b. neutralization
    c. thio
    d. ion
    _____

44. All hydroxide relaxers can swell the hair up to:
    a. tenfold its normal diameter
    b. twice its normal diameter
    c. once its normal diameter
    d. three times its diameter
    _____

45. Hydroxide relaxers remove one atom of sulfur from a disulfide bond converting it into a:
    a. lanthionine bond
    b. hydrogen bond
    c. sulfur bond
    d. cross bond
    _____

46. Disulfide bonds broken by hydroxide relaxers can never be:
    a. restretched
    b. re-formed
    c. oxidized
    d. compatible
    _____

47. Hydroxide ions left in the hair after a relaxer can be neutralized using a(n):
    a. acid-balanced shampoo
    b. conditioning rinse
    c. thio neutralizer
    d. acid-free shampoo
    _____

48. Relaxers containing one component used without any additional mixing are:
    a. thio relaxers
    b. neutral relaxers
    c. metal hydroxide relaxers
    d. normalizing relaxers
    _____

49. Sodium hydroxide relaxers (NaOH) are commonly called:
    a. potassium relaxers
    b. lye relaxers
    c. thio relaxers
    d. guanidine relaxers
    _____

50. A relaxer with two components mixed immediately prior to use is:
    a. ammonium hydroxide relaxer
    c. thioglycolate relaxer
    b. guanidine hydroxide relaxer
    d. lithium hydroxide relaxer ____

51. Lithium hydroxide relaxers and potassium hydroxide relaxers are advertised and sold as:
    a. conditioner relaxers
    c. no chemical relaxers
    b. no-lye relaxers
    d. lye relaxers ____

52. Ammonium sulfite and ammonium bisulfite are marketed as:
    a. lanthionization relaxers
    c. no-hydroxide relaxers
    b. mild alternative relaxers
    d. lye relaxers ____

53. Cream used to protect the skin and scalp during a hair-relaxing process is:
    a. neutral cream
    c. coating cream
    b. scalp cream
    d. base cream ____

54. The strength of relaxers is determined by the concentration of:
    a. ammonia
    c. salts
    b. hydroxide
    d. atoms ____

55. To avoid overprocessing during a retouch relaxer application, wait until the last few minutes of processing to apply relaxer to the area:
    a. closest to the midshaft
    c. closest to the sides
    b. closest to the scalp
    d. closest to the front ____

56. Conditioners with an acidic pH that condition and normalize hair prior to shampooing are:
    a. conditioning rinses
    c. normalizing lotions
    b. conditioning shampoos
    d. acid-based relaxers ____

57. Curl re-formation does not straighten the hair, it simply makes the existing curl:
    a. larger and looser
    c. tighter and open
    b. smaller and longer
    d. open and soft ____

58. To avoid scalp irritation, prior to the application of a hydroxide relaxer never:
    a. shampoo the hair
    c. condition the hair
    b. cut the hair
    d. comb the hair ____

59. To avoid excessive stretching of the hair when combing out tangles, use a:
    a. tail comb
    c. wide-toothed comb
    b. plastic comb
    d. barber comb ____

60. Performing texture services involves powerful chemicals that must be handled with:
   a. ease
   b. caution
   c. gloves
   d. disregard _____

61. The term used to describe removing excess water before the application of a neutralizer is:
   a. processing
   b. conditioning
   c. blotting
   d. rinsing _____

62. When checking for test curl development, the test curl should reflect:
   a. loose S formation
   b. firm S formation
   c. small wave
   d. breakage _____

63. When performing test curls, the rod should be unwound approximately:
   a. ½ turn
   b. 1 turn
   c. 1½ turns
   d. 2 full turns _____

64. Incorrect placement of the rubber band of perm rods will cause band marks or:
   a. shrinkage
   b. protection
   c. tension
   d. breakage _____

65. When working with hair that has been chemically relaxed, you should avoid using:
   a. shampoo
   b. shears
   c. hot irons
   d. protective equipment _____

CHAPTER 19—HAIRCOLORING

1. A key factor in determining appropriate haircoloring services is understanding the client's:
   a. age
   b. motivation
   c. service
   d. style ____

2. Once a stylist demonstrates the ability to skillfully color a client's hair, the client will generally:
   a. remain loyal
   b. switch to a different stylist
   c. ask the stylist to remove the haircolor
   d. never return to the salon again ____

3. In choosing hair color for a client, a determining factor is the hair:
   a. natural style
   b. profession
   c. length
   d. structure ____

4. The layer of the hair that provides strength and elasticity is the:
   a. cortex layer
   b. cuticle layer
   c. follicle layer
   d. medulla layer ____

5. The outermost layer of the hair that protects and provides strength is the:
   a. cuticle layer
   b. medulla layer
   c. papilla layer
   d. structure layer ____

6. In individual hair strands, hair texture is determined by the:
   a. cuticle
   b. cortex
   c. diameter
   d. length ____

7. Hair color applied to fine hair may look:
   a. darker
   b. lighter
   c. shorter
   d. dull ____

8. Haircoloring services on coarse-textured hair may take:
   a. faster to process
   b. longer to process
   c. porosity to process
   d. liquids to process ____

9. Hair with a tight cuticle resistant to moisture or chemicals is defined as having:
   a. average porosity
   b. poor porosity
   c. low porosity
   d. porous porosity ____

10. The predominant melanin that gives black or brown color to hair is:
    a. pheomelanin
    b. natural melanin
    c. individual melanin
    d. eumelanin ____

11. Pigment that lies under the natural hair color is the:
   a. contributing pigment
   c. predominant pigment
   b. combination pigment
   d. exposed pigment _____

12. The lightness or darkness of a color is called the:
   a. range
   c. pigment
   b. level
   d. degree _____

13. The system used by colorists to analyze the lightness or darkness of a hair color is the:
   a. measurement system
   c. color system
   b. natural system
   d. level system _____

14. Hair color levels are arranged on a scale from:
   a. 1 to 12
   c. 1 to 5
   b. 1 to 10
   d. 0 to 10 _____

15. Hair color tones can be described as:
   a. warm, neutral, and hot
   c. cool, neutral, and even
   b. warm, neutral, and cool
   d. cool, warm, and primary _____

16. Colors that absorb light and appear darker than their actual level are:
   a. primary colors
   c. warm colors
   b. cool colors
   d. neutral colors _____

17. Warm tones reflect light and may appear:
   a. ash
   c. cool
   b. smokey
   d. lighter _____

18. Colors that are described as sandy or tan are considered:
   a. primary tones
   c. intensity tones
   b. natural tones
   d. formulation tones _____

19. The first step in performing a haircolor service is to identify:
   a. the natural growth pattern
   c. neutral tones
   b. natural levels
   d. intensity tones _____

20. Colors that we see are contained in the:
   a. invisible light spectrum
   c. color formulation
   b. color wheel
   d. visible light spectrum _____

21. Artificial hair colors are developed from the primary and secondary colors that form:
   a. base colors
   c. permanent tones
   b. tonality colors
   d. drastic colors _____

22. A color that will help minimize orange tones in the hair is a:
    a. violet base color   c. secondary color
    b. blue base color   d. gold base color   ____

23. A system that is used to understand color relationships is the:
    a. color wheel   c. law of color
    b. level system   d. primary color system   ____

24. Colors that are pure or fundamental and cannot be achieved
    from a mixture are:
    a. level colors   c. cool colors
    b. secondary colors   d. primary colors   ____

25. The primary colors are:
    a. red, blue, and orange   c. yellow, blue, and red
    b. blue, red, and violet   d. red, yellow, and green   ____

26. The darkest and only cool primary color is:
    a. green   c. red
    b. ash   d. blue   ____

27. Red added to blue-based colors will cause them to appear:
    a. lighter   c. golden
    b. darker   d. yellow   ____

28. A color achieved by mixing a secondary color and its
    neighboring primary color is a:
    a. primary color   c. secondary color
    b. tertiary color   d. base color   ____

29. Equal proportions of primary colors will produce:
    a. neutral   c. black
    b. secondary   d. brighter   ____

30. A secondary color is obtained by mixing equal parts of two:
    a. base colors   c. neutral colors
    b. primary colors   d. cool colors   ____

31. A primary and secondary color positioned opposite each other
    on the color wheel are:
    a. neutralizing colors   c. opposing colors
    b. combination colors   d. complementary colors   ____

32. Complementary colors are used in color formulation to:
    a. oppose together   c. neutralize each other
    b. attract each other   d. highlight each other   ____

33. The process of diffusing natural color pigment or artificial color from the hair is:
    a. hair lightening   c. hair tinting
    b. hair lifting   d. hair colorization   ____

34. All permanent hair color products and lighteners contain an oxidizing agent and a(n):
    a. neutralizing agent   c. alkalizing ingredient
    b. developer ingredient   d. booster agent   ____

35. A hair-lightening process occurs when the alkaline peroxide:
    a. breaks up the primary color c. dissolves the oxidizing agent
    b. breaks up the melanin   d. breaks up the neutral color   ____

36. Temporary color pigment molecules do not penetrate because they are:
    a. weak   c. neutral
    b. soft   d. large   ____

37. Semipermanent hair color on average should last:
    a. 4 to 6 days   c. 8 to 10 weeks
    b. 4 to 6 weeks   d. 5 to 10 weeks   ____

38. Haircoloring that penetrates the hair shaft and is formulated to deposit but not lift color is:
    a. demipermanent hair color c. semipermanent color
    b. permanent hair color   d. semitemporary color   ____

39. Demipermanent hair color is available in a variety of formulas including:
    a. creams, liquid, and sprays c. creams. gels, and liquid
    b. gels, creams, and lotions   d. gels, powders, and sprays   ____

40. Uncolored dye precursors that can be diffused into the hair shaft are used in ;
    a. gel hair color formulas   c. semipermanent hair color formulas
    b. permanent hair color formulas   d. temporary hair color formulas   ____

41. Dye precursors that combine with hydrogen peroxide to form larger tint molecules are:
    a. aniline peroxide   c. base derivatives
    b. aniline derivatives   d. no-ammonia formulas   ____

42. Although many semipermanent and demipermanent colors use alkalizing agents other than ammonia, they are not necessarily any less:
    a. damaging
    b. effective
    c. colorful
    d. durable ____

43. Permanent haircoloring products are mixed with:
    a. no-ammonia
    b. aniline derivates
    c. hydrogen peroxide
    d. dye precursors ____

44. Permanent hair color products used for gray hair remove natural pigment and:
    a. add natural pigment
    b. add artificial color
    c. remove gray hair
    d. add ammonia tint ____

45. To provide maximum lift in a one-process color service, most high-lift colors require:
    a. 20 volume peroxide
    b. 15 volume peroxide
    c. 30 volume peroxide
    d. 40 volume peroxide ____

46. Haircoloring products that change hair color by creating a progressive buildup contain:
    a. henna colors
    b. chemical colors
    c. metallic colors
    d. vegetable colors ____

47. The most common developer used in haircoloring is:
    a. chemical agent
    b. developer strength
    c. hydrogen peroxide
    d. compound agents ____

48. Lighteners are chemical compounds that lighten natural hair pigment by dispersing, dissolving, and:
    a. decreasing
    b. developer
    c. decolorizing
    d. achieving ____

49. When hydrogen peroxide is mixed with a lightener formula, it releases:
    a. volume
    b. oxygen
    c. color
    d. hydrogen ____

50. During the decolorization process, natural hair can go through as many as:
    a. 2 stages
    b. 1 stage
    c. 5 stages
    d. 10 stages ____

51. Toners are used to achieve pale, delicate colors and are applied to create the correct degree of:
    a. unwanted pigment
    b. contributing pigment
    c. gold pigment
    d. desired shade ____

52. The test required by the U.S. Federal Food, Drug and Cosmetic Act to determine client allergies or sensitivities is the:
   a. swab test
   b. process test
   c. strand test
   d. predisposition test ____

53. To determine how hair will react to a selected color formula, perform a(n):
   a. preliminary strand test
   b. predisposition test
   c. allergy test
   d. patch test ____

54. When selecting a semipermanent color, remember that color applied on top of color creates:
   a. a lighter color
   b. a natural color
   c. a darker color
   d. a brighter color ____

55. Permanent hair color applications are classified as double-process or:
   a. lifting processes
   b. single-process
   c. deposit colors
   d. strand processes ____

56. The application process that is used for first-time color applications is:
   a. retouch process
   b. double-process
   c. virgin application
   d. new application ____

57. Overlapping color can cause breakage and create a sign of roots or:
   a. lightening agent
   b. line of demarcation
   c. barrier line
   d. streaking ____

58. Double-process lightening is prelightening hair to a very blonde stage and applying a:
   a. toner
   b. foundation
   c. rinse
   d. bleach ____

59. For a single-process color for virgin hair, the color processes fastest at:
   a. the shaft
   b. the scalp
   c. the ends
   d. the middle ____

60. Cream lighteners are formulated to be used:
   a. with glaze
   b. on the scalp
   c. on the ends
   d. off the scalp ____

61. The three forms of hair lighteners are:
   a. cream, powder, and scalp
   b. oil, cream, and clear
   c. powder, conditioning, and oil
   d. oil, powder, and cream ____

62. An oxidizer added to hydrogen peroxide to increase its lifting power action is a(n):
   a. powder
   b. activator
   c. ion
   d. crystal _____

63. A technique of coloring strands of hair darker than the natural color is:
   a. highlighting
   b. double-process
   c. tinting
   d. lowlighting _____

64. A foil technique where a straight and narrow section of hair at the scalp is positioned for color or lightener application is:
   a. the cap technique
   b. slicing
   c. weaving
   d. lowlights _____

65. In the foil technique when selected strands are picked up from a narrow section of hair with a zigzag motion of the comb, and lightener is applied in:
   a. slicing
   b. baliage
   c. free-form technique
   d. weaving _____

66. When coloring for a client with 80 to 100 percent gray, the color levels that provide the best coverage are:
   a. level 8 or lighter
   b. level 9 or lighter
   c. level 4 and darker
   d. level 7 and darker _____

67. To cover unpigmented hair in a salt-and-pepper client, the color formulation should be:
   a. one level darker than the natural level
   b. two levels lighter than the natural level
   c. one level lighter than the natural level
   d. one shade darker than the desired level _____

68. Pretreating gray or very resistant hair to allow for better penetration is:
   a. formulating
   b. unpigmenting
   c. predisposition
   d. presoftening _____

69. Preparations designed to equal porosity and deposit a base color in one application are:
   a. neutralizers
   b. fillers
   c. stabilizers
   d. conditioners _____

70. To increase the longevity of a professional color service and preserve the health of clients' hair, the stylist should encourage them to use only:
   a. inexpensive products
   b. imported products
   c. professional products
   d. consumer products _____

CHAPTER 20—SKIN DISEASES AND DISORDERS

1. The signs of aging are influenced by factors such as the sun, health habits, lifestyle, and:
   - a. water
   - b. heredity
   - c. vitamins
   - d. oxygen
   _____

2. The percentage of skin aging that is caused by the rays of the sun is approximately:
   - a. 50 to 55 percent
   - b. 60 to 65 percent
   - c. 70 to 75 percent
   - d. 80 to 85 percent
   _____

3. The UV rays of the sun reach the skin in two different forms, which are:
   - a. UVA and UVB rays
   - b. VBC and ABA rays
   - c. UVA and ULB rays
   - d. UVB and ABB rays
   _____

4. The UVA rays that are deep-penetrating and can go through a glass window are:
   - a. sun rays
   - b. aging rays
   - c. light rays
   - d. ultra rays
   _____

5. Wrinkling and sagging of the skin are caused by weakening collagen fibers and:
   - a. protein fibers
   - b. tissue fibers
   - c. elastin fibers
   - d. dermis fibers
   _____

6. UVB rays contribute to the body's synthesis of vitamin D and other important:
   - a. absorption
   - b. minerals
   - c. elements
   - d. rejuvenation
   _____

7. Daily moisturizers or protective lotions should have a sunscreen with an SPF of at least:
   - a. 5
   - b. 8
   - c. 10
   - d. 15
   _____

8. The American Cancer Society checklist used to recognize skin cancer is:
   - a. asymmetry, big, colored, diameter
   - b. border, color, diameter, evolving
   - c. angle, border, continued, diameter
   - d. asymmetry, border, color, diameter
   _____

9. A salon should not service a client who is suffering from a(n):
   - a. skin condition
   - b. inflamed skin disorder
   - c. skin discoloration
   - d. pustule
   _____

10. A small circumscribed elevation of the skin that contains no fluid but may develop pus is a:
    a. macula
    b. scar
    c. mole
    d. papule _____

11. An abnormal cell mass resulting from excessive multiplication of cells and varying in size, shape, and color is a:
    a. tumor
    b. mole
    c. macula
    d. bulla _____

12. A crack in the skin that penetrates the dermis is a:
    a. split
    b. crust
    c. pustule
    d. fissure _____

13. Keratin-filled cysts that appear just under the epidermis and have no visible openings are:
    a. milia
    b. ulcers
    c. crust
    d. pustules _____

14. Any thin plate of dry or oily epidermal flakes in the scalp area is referred to as:
    a. scales
    b. dandruff
    c. flakes
    d. comedo _____

15. Sebum from a comedo exposed to the environment turns black and:
    a. closes
    b. opens
    c. oxidizes
    d. removes _____

16. Comedones should be removed under aseptic conditions using proper:
    a. skin lotions
    b. extraction procedures
    c. electric tools
    d. skin conditioners _____

17. A chronic skin condition characterized by inflammation of the sebaceous glands is:
    a. freckles
    b. acne
    c. tumors
    d. milia _____

18. An inflammation of the sebaceous glands characterized by dry or oily crusting or itchiness is:
    a. seborrheic dermatitis
    b. seborrheic acne
    c. sebaceous masses
    d. bacterium acne _____

19. A dry, scaly skin condition due to a deficiency or absence of sebum caused by old age or exposure to the cold is:
    a. cystic
    b. cortisone
    c. rosacea
    d. asteatosis _____

20. A disorder of the sweat gland caused by excessive exposure to the heat is:
    a. steatoma
    b. miliaria rubra
    c. anhidrosis
    d. dermatitis
    _____

21. A painful itching skin disease with dry or moist lesions that a physician needs to treat is:
    a. eczema
    b. acne
    c. psoriasis
    d. cyst
    _____

22. A contagious recurring viral infection characterized by blisters on the lips or nostrils is:
    a. eczema simplex
    b. macula simplex
    c. herpes simplex
    d. contact dermatitis
    _____

23. The medical term for abnormal skin inflammation is:
    a. abrasion
    b. dermatitis
    c. psoriasis
    d. bulla
    _____

24. Prolonged or repeated direct skin contact with chemicals has the potential to cause:
    a. allergic reactions
    b. histamine reactions
    c. keloids
    d. absorption
    _____

25. The chemicals released by the immune system to enlarge the vessels around an injury are:
    a. correctors
    b. irritants
    c. allergens
    d. histamines
    _____

26. Surprisingly, a very common salon irritant is:
    a. soap
    b. air
    c. tap water
    d. shampoo
    _____

27. Abnormal brown or wine-colored skin discoloration with a circular and irregular shape is a:
    a. mole
    b. stain
    c. chloasma
    d. lentigo
    _____

28. The absence of melanin pigment from the body and skin sensitivity to light are signs of:
    a. nevus
    b. lentignes
    c. asteatosis
    d. albinism
    _____

29. A spot or blemish spot on the skin that requires medical attention if there is a change is a:
    a. blemish
    b. mole
    c. freckle
    d. keratoma
    _____

30. The most common type of skin cancer characterized by light or pearly nodules is:
   a. basal cell carcinoma
   b. malignant melanoma
   c. squamous cell melanoma
   d. verruca cell

   ____

CHAPTER 21—HAIR REMOVAL

1. Hair removal approaches fall into two major categories, which are:
   a. laser and waxing
   b. temporary and permanent
   c. waxing and tweezing
   d. permanent and semipermanent
   _____

2. Terms that refer to the overgrowth of hair on the body are hypertrichosis and:
   a. excessive
   b. hypersensitive
   c. hirsuties
   d. downy
   _____

3. During the client consultation, all clients should complete a questionnaire that discloses skin disorders, allergies, and:
   a. medications
   b. topicals
   c. diet
   d. assessments
   _____

4. One of the main purposes of a client consultation is to determine the presence of any:
   a. density
   b. follicles
   c. electrolysis
   d. contraindications
   _____

5. The removal of hair with electrical current that destroys the growth cells of the hair is:
   a. photoepilation
   b. electrolysis
   c. electromagnetic
   d. laser
   _____

6. Intense light therapy used to destroy the growth cells of the hair follicles is:
   a. photoepilation
   b. epilation
   c. electrolysis
   d. depilation
   _____

7. A rapid method of removing hair with the use of beams pulsed on the skin is:
   a. laser hair removal
   b. electromagnetic
   c. electrolysis
   d. photobeams
   _____

8. An absolute requirement for laser hair removal is that the hair being removed must be:
   a. lighter than the surrounding skin
   b. darker than the surrounding skin
   c. administered to the surrounding skin
   d. removed slowly
   _____

9. In the nape area, the most common form of hair removal is usually performed using electric:
   a. tweezers
   b. clippers
   c. shears
   d. lasers
   _____

10. A positive impact on the overall attractiveness of the face can be achieved with:
    a. evenly spaced eyes
    b. client consultation
    c. client's wishes
    d. correctly shaped eyebrows _____

11. The natural arch of the eyebrow follows the:
    a. orbital bone
    b. frontal bone
    c. mandible bone
    d. frontal muscle _____

12. A term used to describe unwanted hair is:
    a. downy hair
    b. lanugo hair
    c. papilla
    d. superfluous hair _____

13. Electronic tweezers transmit radio frequency energy into the follicle area, dehydrating and eventually destroying the:
    a. cuticle
    b. cortex
    c. lanugo
    d. papilla _____

14. A caustic substance used for the temporary removal of superfluous hair at the skin level is:
    a. a cold wax
    b. a photoepilation
    c. a depilatory
    d. electric tweezers _____

15. The product composition of cold and hot wax is primarily beeswax and:
    a. aloe gel
    b. resins
    c. sugar
    d. caustic _____

16. Disposable gloves should be worn during a waxing service to prevent contact with possible:
    a. inflamed skin
    b. sensitive skin
    c. previously treated skin
    d. bloodborne pathogens _____

17. Wax should never be applied over warts, moles, abrasions, or:
    a. irritated or inflamed skin
    b. dark or red areas
    c. freckles
    d. scaly skin _____

18. To prevent wax contamination, an applicator should be placed in the wax:
    a. twice
    b. once
    c. when needed
    d. often _____

19. In a waxing treatment, the wax should be applied:
    a. against the hair growth
    b. in the excessive amounts required
    c. in the direction of the hair growth
    d. in the treated areas _____

20. An epilator treatment that involves using a thick-based product appropriate for sensitive skin is:
    a. beeswax
    b. sugaring
    c. cold wax
    d. depilatory _____

21. Apply pressure to remove a fabric waxing strip and pull:
    a. straight up
    b. in the direction of hair growth
    c. downward
    d. in the opposite direction of hair growth _____

22. To prevent skin irritation or burns, the temperature of wax should be tested:
    a. on the client's skin
    b. prior to application
    c. after the application
    d. during the application _____

23. A temporary hair removal method practiced in many Eastern cultures is the process of:
    a. threading
    b. tattooing
    c. removal
    d. laser _____

24. If redness or swelling occurs after a waxing treatment, soothe the skin with the application of:
    a. aloe gel
    b. lotion
    c. disinfectant
    d. astringent _____

25. A wax that is thick and does not require fabric strips for removal is:
    a. aloe wax
    b. cold wax
    c. honey wax
    d. chemical wax _____

CHAPTER 22—FACIALS

1. The preliminary parts of a facial treatment that determine the treatments to be performed are:
   a. skin consultation and payment
   b. skin analysis and consultation
   c. client consultation and draping
   d. skin analysis and product choice ____

2. The health screening performed prior to a facial treatment is used by the technician to determine any:
   a. product preference   c. financial background
   b. client lifestyle   d. contraindications ____

3. Clients with obvious skin abnormalities such as open sores, fever blisters, or abnormal-looking signs should be:
   a. advised of services   c. referred to a physician
   b. provided treatments   d. provided free services ____

4. When removing a cleanser from the eye area, it should be removed with damp facial sponges or cotton pads:
   a. in an upward and outward movement
   b. in down and across movements
   c. with friction movements
   d. in upward and across movements ____

5. When performing a skin analysis with a magnifying lamp, the first thing the technician should look for is the presence or absence of:
   a. skin types   c. evaporated cells
   b. visible pores   d. oily skin areas ____

6. If the client is not producing enough sebum, the skin type is characterized as:
   a. clean   c. alipidic
   b. oily   d. normal ____

7. Skin that has small pores and may be flaky or dry with fine lines and wrinkles is characterized as:
   a. dehydrated   c. normal
   b. oily   d. sensitive ____

8. Oily skin or skin that produces too much sebum may appear shiny or greasy and have:
   a. dead cells   c. flakes
   b. small pores   d. large pores ____

9. Pores that are clogged from dead cells building up in the follicle may have the appearance of open:
   a. creams
   c. milia
   b. comedones
   d. sebum
   ____

10. The difference between closed and open comedones is the size of the follicle opening or the:
    a. gland
    c. ostium
    b. sebum
    d. skin
    ____

11. When the follicle becomes clogged, resulting in an infection of the follicle, it is caused by a type of acne bacteria called:
    a. hydrators
    c. sebum imbalance
    b. anaerobic
    d. hyperpigmentation
    ____

12. Red pimples that do not have a pus head are referred to as:
    a. elastin pimples
    c. acne pigmentation
    b. acne papules
    d. acne oxygen
    ____

13. A skin condition caused by sun exposure or hormone imbalances resulting in dark blotches of color in areas of the skin is:
    a. hypertrichosis
    c. dehydration
    b. hydrators
    d. hyperpigmentation
    ____

14. A chronic hereditary disorder indicated by constant or frequent facial blushing is:
    a. rosacea
    c. pustules
    b. tinea
    d. comedones
    ____

15. A nonfoaming cleansing product that is designed to cleanse dry and sensitive skin is:
    a. astringent lotion
    c. foaming cleanser
    b. cleansing powder
    d. cleansing milk
    ____

16. Cleansing products that foam and rinse off easily generally contain surfactants also known as:
    a. astringents
    c. detergents
    b. skin toners
    d. exfoliants
    ____

17. Skin products designed to lower the pH of skin after cleansing and remove excess cleansing product are fresheners, astringents, or:
    a. detergents
    c. toners
    b. surfactants
    d. emollients
    ____

18. Exfoliant products are used on skin surfaces to make the skin look smoother by:
a. removing excess moisture
b. removing excess dead cells
c. removing makeup
d. adding moisture to skin

_____

19. Cosmetology professionals are only allowed to use products that remove surface dead cells from the:
a. internal dermis
b. stratum corneum
c. stratum dermis
d. dermal layer

_____

20. A gentle chemical exfoliation acid that helps dissolve the bonds and intercellular cement between cells is:
a. alpha hydroxy acid
b. emulsion acid
c. astringent acid
d. steaming acid

_____

21. A salon-type of alpha hydroxy acid exfoliant that contains a concentration of 20 to 30 percent acid is referred to as a:
a. skin brushing
b. peel
c. beta hydroxy acid
d. removal

_____

22. A chemical exfoliant that works by dissolving keratin protein in the surface skin cells is known as an enzyme peel or:
a. keratolytic
b. salt peel
c. cream treatment
d. tonic peel

_____

23. An enzyme cream-type skin peel that forms a crust and is rolled off the skin is a:
a. papain
b. scrubbing
c. emulsion
d. gommage

_____

24. Moisturizers that increase the water content of the skin's surface with a product that is water-binding are known as:
a. toners
b. astringents
c. hydrators
d. emollients

_____

25. A fatty or oily ingredient used to block moisture from leaving the skin is a(n):
a. emollient
b. exfoliant
c. toner
d. sunscreen

_____

26. Clients should be advised to use sunscreens that protect against both UVA and:
a. VBB sun rays
b. UVB sun rays
c. UTB sun rays
d. ATB sun rays

_____

27. Highly concentrated skin products applied under a moisturizer or sunscreen are:
   a. serums
   b. tonics
   c. masks
   d. shielding _____

28. Lubricants applied to the face to make the skin slippery during a treatment are:
   a. exfoliant creams
   b. massage creams
   c. AHA
   d. clay masks _____

29. Soothing masks that have antibacterial ingredients and are helpful for acne-prone skin are:
   a. water based
   b. medicated based
   c. moisture based
   d. clay based _____

30. Masks that do not dry the skin and often contain oils and emollients as well as humectants are:
   a. oil masks
   b. gel masks
   c. cream masks
   d. serums _____

31. Paraffin used as a mask has no skin benefit unless mixed with a(n):
   a. exfoliating cream
   b. treatment cream
   c. oxygen cream
   d. massage treatment _____

32. A plaster-like mask that, when mixed with water, causes a chemical reaction is known as a(n):
   a. clay mask
   b. alginate mask
   c. quick mask
   d. modelage mask _____

33. The thin, open-meshed, woven cotton fabric used in the penetration of the mask application is:
   a. plastic
   b. silk
   c. gauze
   d. satin _____

34. The term used to describe the manual or mechanical manipulation of the body is:
   a. friction
   b. massage
   c. movements
   d. circulation _____

35. To master massage techniques, the cosmetologist should have a basic working knowledge of:
   a. anatomy and physiology
   b. costs of products
   c. skin toners
   d. gommage _____

36. The direction of movement in massage techniques should always be from the insertion of the muscle:
   a. toward the end
   b. behind the muscle
   c. toward its origin
   d. at the motor point _____

108

37. The massage movement that is a light continuous stroking movement with the fingers in a slow rhythmic manner is:
    a. tapotement   c. kneading
    b. petrissage   d. effleurage   ____

38. The kneading massage movement performed by lifting, squeezing, and pressing the tissue with light, firm pressure is:
    a. petrissage   c. effleurage
    b. rolling   d. stroking   ____

39. The deep rubbing of friction massage movements on the skin has been known to have a significant effect on the:
    a. texture and appearance of dry skin
    c. activity and texture of the skin
    b. circulation and glandular activity of the skin
    d. underlying structure activity of the skin   ____

40. The most stimulating type of massage that should be performed using extreme care and discretion is:
    a. fulling   c. tapotement
    b. stroking   d. chucking   ____

41. The point on the skin over the muscle where pressure and stimulation will cause contraction of the muscle is referred to as the:
    a. insertion point   c. origin point
    b. motor point   d. connection point   ____

42. A significant benefit of a facial steamer that heats and produces steam is that the steam produced will soften and relax:
    a. dry skin conditions   c. follicle accumulations
    b. oily skin conditions   d. the client   ____

43. When using the brushing machine to perform an exfoliation, the skin should be treated with a(n):
    a. thin layer of cleanser or moisturizer
    b. fairly thick layer of cleanser or moisturizer
    c. face freshener
    d. astringent lotion   ____

44. The skin suction and cold spray machine is used to increase circulation and should be used only on nonsensitive or:
    a. oily skin   c. mature skin
    b. hydrated skin   d. noninflamed skin   ____

45. The use of electric currents to treat the skin is a form of:
    a. electrotherapy   c. cold spray therapy
    b. magnetic therapy   d. microfarad therapy ____

46. The process of softening and emulsifying hardened sebum stuck in the follicles is called:
    a. massage therapy   c. desincrustation
    b. passive therapy   d. shock treatments   ____

47. Water-soluble products are penetrated into the skin using galvanic current and a process called:
    a. penetration   c. active anode
    b. iontophoresis   d. extraction   ____

48. A galvanic treatment using a computerized device to tone skin and produce a lifting effect on aging skin is:
    a. microcurrent   c. galvanic imaging
    b. microwaves   d. Tesla currents   ____

49. The therapeutic use of essential oils to enhance a person's physical and emotional well-being is:
    a. retailing   c. antidepressants
    b. consultations   d. aromatherapy   ____

50. After the first treatment, every new client should be provided with a thorough consultation that consists of salon treatment programs, education, and:
    a. positive effects   c. proper home care
    b. verbal instructions d. prescription medication ____

1. A base makeup that is used to cover or even out the coloring of skin is:
   - a. blush
   - b. roll-on
   - c. foundation
   - d. cream
   ____

2. Foundation bases are available in stick, cream, mineral powder, and:
   - a. foam
   - b. roll-on
   - c. tint
   - d. liquid
   ____

3. Natural derived pigments or color agents added to foundations to provide color are:
   - a. lakes
   - b. minerals
   - c. emollients
   - d. liquids
   ____

4. The recommended foundation for light coverage on oily to combination skin is:
   - a. water based
   - b. oil free
   - c. cream foundations
   - d. natural foundations
   ____

5. Foundations that provide a heavier base coverage for dry skin are:
   - a. water-based foundations
   - b. cream foundations
   - c. powder-type foundations
   - d. tinted base foundations
   ____

6. Foundation should be blended using:
   - a. lint-free tissues
   - b. disposable makeup sponge
   - c. cotton cloths
   - d. professional brush
   ____

7. Concealers that are used to hide dark circles and imperfections contain talc or:
   - a. tint
   - b. oil
   - c. pigment
   - d. silicone
   ____

8. To keep pressed powder in a cake form, it is usually blended with:
   - a. mineral oil
   - b. binding agents
   - c. scented particles
   - d. cornstarch agents
   ____

9. A makeup product primarily used to add a natural glow to the cheek or face area is a:
   - a. blush
   - b. foundation
   - c. concealer
   - d. highlight
   ____

10. Generally, a darker shade of eye color makes the natural color of the iris appear:
    a. darker
    b. closer
    c. lighter
    d. neutral
    ____

11. Color applied over the eye area to even out skin tones and provide a smooth surface for the blending of other colors is a:
    a. neutral color
    b. contour color
    c. medium color
    d. base color
    ____

12. A color in any finish that deepens and darkens the skin tone and minimizes a specific area is a:
    a. desired color
    b. contour color
    c. highlight color
    d. neutral color
    ____

13. To avoid infection in the tear duct or permanent pigmentation of the mucous membrane lining, eye pencils should never be used:
    a. on the outer rim of eyes
    b. near the lash area
    c. on the inner rim of eyes
    d. on the upper lids
    ____

14. A cosmetic preparation used to darken, define, and thicken eyelashes is:
    a. blush
    b. mascara
    c. foundation
    d. eye shadow
    ____

15. To clean professional makeup brushes, a gentle shampoo or brush solvent is used, and the brush is placed into running water with the:
    a. bristles being flat
    b. ferrule pointing upward
    c. ferrule pointing downward
    d. bristles being covered
    ____

16. Colors obtained by mixing equal parts of two primary colors are:
    a. tertiary colors
    b. complementary colors
    c. mixing colors
    d. secondary colors
    ____

17. A primary and secondary color directly opposite each other on the color wheel are:
    a. secondary colors
    b. conflicting colors
    c. complementary colors
    d. primary colors
    ____

18. Three main factors to consider when choosing color for a client are the client's hair color,
    a. eye color, and skin color
    b. eye placement, and skin texture
    c. skin color, and texture
    d. eye color, and results
    ____

19. Colors that are dominated by blues, greens, violets, and blue-reds are classified as:
    a. cool colors
    c. complementary colors
    b. magenta colors
    d. pigment colors _____

20. Skin tones that contain equal amounts of warm and cool colors are considered:
    a. basic skin tones
    c. cool skin tones
    b. neutral skin tones
    d. warm skin tones _____

21. Complementary colors for green eyes are brown-based reds, which include:
    a. green, blue, and silver
    c. taupe, caramel, and peach
    b. copper, plum, and mauve
    d. yellow, reds, and neutrals _____

22. The best type of lighting for color selection in the salon consultation area is:
    a. bright light
    c. fluorescent light
    b. natural light
    d. cool light _____

23. Foundation application should start at the center of the face and blend with:
    a. upward and outside motions
    c. downward and slow motions
    b. outward and fast motions
    d. outward and downward motions _____

24. A basic rule of makeup application is that highlighting emphasizes a feature and shadowing:
    a. minimizes a feature
    c. maximizes a feature
    b. shades a feature
    d. outlines a feature _____

25. The second portion of an oval-shaped type face is measured from the:
    a. hairline to the top of the eyebrows
    b. end of the nose to the bottom of the chin
    c. top of eyebrows to end of nose
    d. side of ears to end of nose _____

26. The facial shape composed of comparatively straight lines, a wide forehead, and square jaw is the:
    a. square-shaped face
    c. oval-shaped face
    b. round-shaped face
    d. diamond-shaped face _____

27. The long, narrow facial shape with greater length in proportion to its width is the:
    a. triangle-shaped face
    c. oblong-shaped face
    b. diamond-shaped face
    d. square-shaped face _____

28. To minimize a short, flat nose, a lighter foundation is applied:
    a. on the cheeks and sides of the nose, ending at the tip
    b. down the center of the nose, ending at the tip
    c. on the sides of the nose and nostrils
    d. onto the sides of the nose and into the laugh lines of the face
    _____

29. To set foundation and prevent the transfer to clothing, use:
    a. darker foundation
    b. translucent powder
    c. natural skin tones
    d. pressed powder
    _____

30. In eyebrow arching, the highest part of an eyebrow arch should be from the outer circle to the:
    a. corner of the eyes
    b. iris of the eye upward
    c. outer corner of the nose
    d. inner corner of the eye upward
    _____

CHAPTER 24—NAIL DISEASES AND DISORDERS

1. A normal healthy nail is firm and flexible and should be
    a. smooth and unspotted
    b. uneven and unspotted
    c. unspotted and long
    d. medium length and unspotted
    _____

2. A nail disorder is classified as a condition that is caused by:
    a. injury or disease
    b. free edge
    c. nail surface
    d. improper care or white spots
    _____

3. If a client has skin that is infected, inflamed, or swollen, the client should be referred to:
    a. a series of nail treatments
    b. a physician
    c. a licensed manicurist
    d. an upscale salon
    _____

4. A condition of the nails in which blood clots form under the nail plate is:
    a. damaged nails
    b. swollen nails
    c. bruised nails
    d. eggshell nails
    _____

5. When performing nail services on a client with nail ridges running vertically down the nail plate, it is recommended that the technician:
    a. carefully remove the nail plate
    b. carefully buff the nail plate
    c. refuse to service the client
    d. refer the client to a medical doctor
    _____

6. A common nail condition where living skin around the nail splits due to dryness of the skin is:
    a. beau's lines
    b. leukonychia spots
    c. onych
    d. hangnails
    _____

7. A localized area of increased pigment cells within the matrix bed is responsible for the nail condition:
    a. beau's lines
    b. agnail
    c. melanonychia
    d. melanin
    _____

8. A common term used to describe a nail with a highly curved nail plate is:
    a. bitten nail
    b. split nail
    c. bruised nail
    d. plicatured nail
    _____

9. An abnormal nail condition that is the result of damage to the eponychium or hyponychium and occurs when skin is stretched by the nail plate is:
   a. nail pterygium
   b. curved nails
   c. pincer nail
   d. nail cuticle
   _____

10. Parasites that under some conditions may cause infection to the feet and hands are:
    a. fungi
    b. pusd.
    c. pincer
    mold
    _____

11. Nail fungi are of concern to the salon because they can be transmitted through unsanitary implements and are:
    a. unhealthy
    b. fragile
    c. contagious
    d. viruses
    _____

12. A term that should not be used when referring to infections of the fingernails or toenails is:
    a. tinea
    b. bacteria
    c. mold
    d. pathogens
    _____

13. To prevent fungal organisms on the nail, in addition to the sanitation and disinfection of implements, the technician must properly:
    a. clean and prepare the natural nail plate
    b. clean and prepare the nail cuticle area
    c. remove nail polish remover from nails
    d. file nails with a disposable file
    _____

14. A typical bacterial infection on the nail plate can be identified in the early stages as a:
    a. blue-black spot under the nail
    b. yellow-green spot on the nail
    c. white spot on the nail bed
    d. black spots on the nail plate
    _____

15. To avoid the spread of any nail diseases or bacterial infections, it is imperative that the technician use:
    a. strict sanitation and disinfection practices
    b. familiar sanitation practices
    c. strict disinfection and proficient skill techniques
    d. low-level sanitation and disinfection practices
    _____

16. The lifting of the nail plate from the bed without shedding is a nail disease called:
    a. onycholysis
    b. onychomadesis
    c. nail psoriasis
    d. ingrown nails
    _____

17. A bacterial inflammation surrounding the nail tissue that may be the result of excessive exposure to water is:
    a. paronychia
    c. salmon patches
    b. tinea pedis
    d. pyogenic
    ____

18. The medical term for fungal infections associated with the feet is:
    a. tinea pathogenic
    c. tinea alopecia
    b. tinea pedis
    d. paronychia
    ____

19. The technical term used to describe bitten nails is:
    a. onychophagy
    c. onycholysis
    b. onychorrhexis
    d. onyx
    ____

20. The naturally occurring skin bacteria that can grow out of control and cause an infection if conditions are correct is:
    a. melanonychia
    c. leukonychia
    b. pseudomonas aeruginosa
    d. pterygium
    ____

CHAPTER 25—MANICURING

1. A manicuring table lamp should have an incandescent bulb with wattage no higher than:
   a. 10 to 30 watts
   c. 70 to 90 watts
   b. 40 to 60 watts
   d. 100 to 120 watts
   ____

2. Disinfection containers for manicure implements should be large enough for implements to be:
   a. partially immersed
   c. completely immersed
   b. removed with hands
   d. completely cleaned
   ____

3. Lids are required on disinfectant containers to prevent:
   a. spilling
   c. immersion
   b. contamination
   d. sharing
   ____

4. Manicuring implements should be placed in the disinfectant container after being:
   a. used several times
   c. properly marked
   b. used by the client
   d. properly cleaned
   ____

5. A wooden pusher used to remove cuticle tissue is disposable and should be:
   a. sanitized and reused
   c. placed in a cabinet drawer
   b. discarded after each use
   d. washed with soap and water
   ____

6. A metal pusher is used to push back the eponychium and gently scrape cuticle tissue from the:
   a. natural nail root
   c. nail free edge
   b. natural nail plate
   d. nail matrix
   ____

7. Fine grit abrasives are designed for removing very fine scratches and:
   a. buffing and polishing
   c. beveling the nail
   b. aggressive buffing
   d. reducing nail length
   ____

8. To bevel a nail, use gentle pressure and angle the file with a:
   a. 60-degree angle
   c. 45-degree angle
   b. 90-degree angle
   d. straight angle
   ____

9. Clean abrasives or implements stored in plastic bags or sealed airtight containers promote:
   a. air circulation
   c. storage problems
   b. bacterial growth
   d. ineffective storage
   ____

10. A nipper should be used to carefully trim away the:
    a. nail plate
    c. cuticle area
    b. nail free edge
    d. tags of dead skin
    ____

11. A buffer that shines the nail plate without the use of dry buffing powder is a(n):
   a. abrasive buffer   c. three-way buffer
   b. wooden pusher   d. electric dryer   ____

12. A tool used to shorten the length of the natural nail plate is a(n):
   a. electric dryer   c. nail clipper
   b. wooden pusher   d. nail nipper   ____

13. The time necessary to properly clean and disinfect implements after each use is:
   a. 10 minutes   c. 60 minutes
   b. 20 minutes   d. 30 minutes   ____

14. Brushes used in products that do not harbor the growth of pathogens are considered:
   a. renewable brushes   c. bacteria free
   b. self-disinfecting   d. self-cleaning   ____

15. Small fiber-free squares used to apply or remove product are:
   a. cotton   c. fibers
   b. linen   d. pledgets   ____

16. Nail products should be removed from their containers using a:
   a. plastic or metal spatula   c. plastic or metal brush
   b. finger   d. cotton   ____

17. Cosmetic products containing a high water content provide the growth opportunity for:
   a. pathogens   c. fibers
   b. containers   d. vapors   ____

18. The use of bar soap is not recommended as it may:
   a. be expensive   c. harbor bacteria
   b. be inexpensive   d. spread ethyl   ____

19. When removing nail polish from wrap-type nail enhancements, use a solvent that is:
   a. acetone   c. quick
   b. non-acetone   d. conditioning   ____

20. Removers that are used to dissolve and remove polish contain solvents of ethyl acetate or:
   a. mineral oil   c. acetone
   b. sodium   d. potassium   ____

21. A product designed to loosen and dissolve dead tissue from the nail plate is:
    a. moisturizing lotion   c. polish remover
    b. nonacetone remover   d. cuticle remover   ____

22. A product designed to improve adhesion of polish to the natural nail is a:
    a. top coat   c. reinforcing coat
    b. nail hardener   d. base coat   ____

23. Nail hardeners that cause adverse reactions to skin may contain:
    a. formaldehyde   c. acrylic
    b. resins   d. dimethyl urea   ____

24. Product information including safe handling, first aid, and proper storage is required in:
    a. Manufacturers Direction Sheets
    b. Material Supply Order Forms
    c. Material Safety Data Sheets
    d. Material Disposal Sheets   ____

25. Generally, it is recommended that the shape of the nail plate enhances the overall:
    a. shape of the cuticle   c. length of the nail
    b. shape of the fingertip   d. shape of the hands   ____

26. The five basic nail shapes are:
    a. square, pointed, oval, flat, and slender
    c. square, squoval, round, pointed, and oval
    b. slender, oval, squoval, square, and pointed
    d. pointed, square, narrow, round, and strong   ____

27. Should a client be accidentally cut and blood drawn, the first precautionary step is to:
    a. put on gloves and inform client
    b. clean with antiseptic solution
    c. stanch bleeding with pressure
    d. discard used materials   ____

28. The three individual procedures for a basic manicure should include:
    a. pre-service, post-service, and disinfection procedures
    b. pre-service, actual service, and post-service
    c. consultation, pre-service, and service performed
    d. pre-service, post-service, and recommendations   ____

29. Success in nail polish application is achieved by using four coats including:
   a. one base coat, one polish color, and two top coats
   b. two polish color, one top coat, and one sealer coat
   c. one base coat, two polish color, and one top coat
   d. one base coat, one polish color, and two top coats ____

30. Massage manipulations should be executed using:
   a. fast rubbing movements
   b. rhythmic and smooth movements
   c. fast, pulsating movements
   d. fast, rotating movements ____

31. The massage movement where the technician holds the client's wrist and bends it back and forth slowly is a form of:
   a. joint movement
   b. circular movement
   c. rotating movement
   d. palm effleurage ____

32. Vigorous joint massage should not be performed if a client has a joint injury or:
   a. arthritis
   b. psoriasis
   c. migraines
   d. artificial nails ____

33. Sitting or working in uncomfortable, strained positions can lead to back, neck, or shoulder injuries and result in:
   a. temporary trauma
   b. carpal tunnel trauma disorders
   c. temporary relaxation
   d. cumulative trauma ____

34. Spa manicures encompass extensive knowledge of nail care and:
   a. skin care treatments
   b. consultations
   c. towel applications
   d. lotion applications ____

35. Spa manicures include massage and skin exfoliation for polishing, smoothing, and enhancing:
   a. massage ambiance
   b. oily cosmetics
   c. professional product penetration
   d. client's preference for cosmetics ____

CHAPTER 26—PEDICURING

1. Pedicure procedures include trimming, shaping, and polishing toenails; exfoliating skin; and:
   a. foot masques
   b. foot massage services
   c. nail plate dissolvers
   d. recommending hair
   _____

2. To ensure healthy, happy feet, professional pedicure services should be performed:
   a. yearly
   b. weekly
   c. monthly
   d. daily
   _____

3. A pedicure tool used to exfoliate dry skin or smooth calluses is a:
   a. rasp
   b. paddle
   c. curette
   d. clipper
   _____

4. A pedicuring station should include a comfortable chair for the client, a footrest for the client, and a(n):
   a. designer chair for the nail professional
   b. designed stool for the client
   c. ergonomic stool for the nail professional
   d. ergonomic chair for the nail professional
   _____

5. To be effective in a pedicure bath, liquid soaps should contain a(n):
   a. scented oil
   b. antibacterial soap
   c. mild detergent
   d. strong detergent
   _____

6. Lotions, oils, and creams are used to condition and moisturize feet and for:
   a. performing a foot massage
   b. disinfecting the foot spa
   c. applying polish to the toenails
   d. removing polish from the toenails
   _____

7. A metal file that is designed to be used in a specific fashion is a:
   a. board
   b. brush
   c. curette
   d. rasp
   _____

8. The tool used to exfoliate dry skin or smooth calluses during a pedicure service is a:
   a. foot bath
   b. foot file
   c. pedicure clipper
   d. toe separator
   _____

9. When working on the foot, it should be grasped between the thumb and fingers at the:
   a. bottom of the foot
   b. heel area
   c. mid-tarsal area
   d. ankle area
   _____

10. The actual pedicure procedure has five basic steps: the soak, nail care, skin care,
    a. polish, and rebook
    b. massage, and polish
    c. massage, and waxing
    d. polish, and exfoliating
    _____

11. When performing a pedicure, apply a firm grip on the client's foot to:
    a. produce a tickling sensation
    b. calm the client
    c. waste finger motions
    d. lock the ankle area
    _____

12. When clipping toenails, extra care should be exercised to avoid breaking the:
    a. hyponychium
    b. dermis
    c. pressure point
    d. elastin
    _____

13. To properly disinfect a foot spa after each pedicure service, the nail technician is required to perform the following steps:
    a. Drain and remove water and contaminants, add more soap and water, and use.
    b. Drain and remove water and contaminants, clean surface, disinfect with approved disinfectant, rinse, and dry.
    c. Drain and remove water, disinfect with approved disinfectant, rinse, and dry.
    d. Change water, add soap , disinfect with approved disinfectant, thoroughly rinse, and dry.
    _____

14. The procedure for cleaning a foot spa at the end of the day is: remove and clean screen of trapped debris, wash screen and inlet and totally immerse in approved disinfectant, then:
    a. flush system with warm water for 5 minutes, rinse, and air dry
    b. rinse out system with warm water for 2 minutes, rinse with cold water, and dry with sponge
    c. flush system with low-sudsing soap and water for 10 minutes, rinse, drain, and air-dry
    d. rinse system with low-sudsing soap and water for 5 minutes, rinse, drain, and towel dry
    _____

15. The weekly maintenance procedure for foot spas requires the disinfectant solution to remain in the foot spa at least:
    a. 4 to 5 hours
    b. 6 to 10 hours
    c. 1 or 2 hours
    d. 2 to 3 hours
    _____

16. Foot massage performed correctly is relaxing to the client, is therapeutic, and:
    a. stimulates nail growth
    b. increases foot pressure
    c. stimulates muscle growth
    d. stimulates blood flow   _____

17. The massage movement used to stretch the muscles and tendons is:
    a. petrissage
    b. effleurage
    c. tapping
    d. kneading   _____

18. A product that should never be placed in the foot bath with the client's feet is a:
    a. solution
    b. antiseptic
    c. magnesium salt
    d. disinfectant   _____

19. Creams or lotions used to help in the removal and smoothing of dry, flaky skin and calluses are:
    a. massage preparations
    b. natural oils
    c. abrasive scrubs
    d. moisturized agents   _____

20. Alkaline cuticle removers should never be applied to:
    a. resins and adhesives
    b. living skin
    c. massage oil products
    d. nail polish   _____

21. Professional strength callus softener products usually contain sodium hydroxide or:
    a. lactic acid
    b. sodium chloride
    c. hydrogen peroxide
    d. mineral clays   _____

22. A hot paraffin bath should not be provided to a client with:
    a. seasonal allergies
    b. diabetic-related problems
    c. vitamin deficiency
    d. premature aging   _____

23. A small "ice cream scooper"-shaped implement used for efficient removal of debris from nail folds and cuticle area is a:
    a. nipper
    b. clipper
    c. curette
    d. spatula   _____

24. Toenail clippers used for a pedicure service should have:
    a. double edges
    b. fairly fine points
    c. fairly straight edges
    d. two even edges   _____

25. Nail rasps are a tool specifically designed to file:
    a. in several directions
    b. across nail grooves
    c. along edges
    d. in one direction   _____

1. Plastic, premolded forms adhered to natural nails to add length or support nail enhancement products are:
   a. nail wraps
   b. nail tips
   c. nail overlays
   d. nail adhesives _____

2. Nail tips break easily without the reinforcement called a(n):
   a. overlay
   b. adhesive
   c. full-well
   d. activator _____

3. A rough surface tool used to shape, smooth, and remove the surface shine on a nail is a(n):
   a. emery board
   b. shine remover
   c. gel activator
   d. abrasive board _____

4. The term used to describe the thickness of nail adhesives is:
   a. strength
   b. viscosity
   c. durability
   d. safety _____

5. Nail tips should never cover more than:
   a. one-half of the nail plate
   b. all the nail plate
   c. one-third of the natural nail plate
   d. tip of natural nail _____

6. The shallow depression area of a nail tip is the:
   a. well
   b. contact
   c. applicator
   d. gelled _____

7. When placing nail tips on the natural nail plate, the technique used is:
   a. stop, hold, and release
   b. stop, rock, and hold
   c. rock, hold, and free
   d. rock, slide, and release _____

8. When blending a nail tip at the contact area, the fine-grit buff block should be held:
   a. at a 45-degree angle against the nail plate
   b. at a right angle against the nail plate
   c. deep into the nail plate
   d. flat across the surface of the nail plate _____

9. The action used with a wooden pusher to remove softened nail tips is:
   a. pull gently with pusher
   b. slide off with clippers
   c. slide off with pusher
   d. nip off with nippers _____

10. Nail enhancements using nail-size pieces of cloth or paper bonded to the nail plate are:
    a. nail wraps
    b. gel nails
    c. adhesive wraps
    d. opaque wraps _____

11. The strongest material used as a nail wrap is:
    a. silk
    b. paper
    c. fiberglass
    d. linen
    _____

12. A product that accelerates the curing process of resins and adhesives is a(n):
    a. heat spike
    b. extender tip
    c. activator
    d. plastic strip
    _____

13. A product applied to the surface of natural nails to remove moisture and improve adhesion is a:
    a. nail blender
    b. nail activator
    c. nail adhesive
    d. nail dehydrator
    _____

14. When applying nail wraps, to prevent the transfer of oil and debris from the technician to the client, use:
    a. gloves
    b. flexible plastic sheets
    c. wooden spatulas
    d. small pieces of cotton
    _____

15. Nail wraps should be rebalanced with resin and new fabric after:
    a. 6 weeks
    b. 8 weeks
    c. 4 weeks
    d. 2 months
    _____

16. A fabric piece cut to completely cover a crack or break in a nail wrap is a:
    a. stress strip
    b. repair patch
    c. rebalance batch
    d. refill strip
    _____

17. A gel-like material that requires an activator to cure is:
    a. gel light application
    b. no-cure gel application
    c. resin gel application
    d. no-light gel application
    _____

18. The improper use of activators can cause a heat spike to the client and:
    a. polymer damage
    b. pulling sensation
    c. surface shine
    d. nail bed damage
    _____

19. To avoid damaging nail wraps when removing existing polish, use a(n):
    a. acetone remover
    b. oil accelerator
    c. resin softener
    d. nonacetone remover
    _____

20. An implement similar to a nail clipper, designed especially for use on nail tips, is a:
    a. tip nipper
    b. tip cutter
    c. stress cutter
    d. tip buffer
    _____

CHAPTER 28—ACRYLIC (METHACRYLATE) NAILS

1. Acrylic (methacrylate) nail enhancements are created by combining monomer liquid with:
    a. monomer powder
    b. polymer powder
    c. liquid powder
    d. molecular powder _____

2. Nail enhancements sculptured with the use of polymer powder are called:
    a. monomer nails
    b. protective nails
    c. synthetic nails
    d. acrylic nails _____

3. Brushes recommended for the application of acrylic (methacrylate) product are:
    a. natural hair
    b. nylon bristles
    c. mixed hair
    d. plastic bristles _____

4. When applying product, the brush is immersed into monomer and the tip of the brush is:
    a. dragged across the surface of the dry polymer powder
    b. pushed gently into the dry polymer powder
    c. immersed into the dry polymer powder
    d. touched to the surface of the dry polymer powder _____

5. As monomer liquid absorbs a polymer powder, the product formed at the tip of the brush is referred to as a:
    a. monomer bead
    b. bead of product
    c. chemical reaction
    d. molded product _____

6. Polymer powder is made using a special chemical reaction called:
    a. polychain
    b. monomer chains
    c. polymerization
    d. methacrylate chains _____

7. In the process of creating acrylic (methacrylate) nails, trillions of monomers are linked together to create:
    a. additives
    b. long chains
    c. dry chemicals
    d. long absorptions _____

8. Additives are responsible for the product durability and color stability of the product, and they ensure:
    a. complete cure or set
    b. complete beads
    c. proper procedure
    d. proper disposal _____

9. Additives used to control the set or curing time in monomer liquids are called:
    a. accelerators and adhesives
    b. controllers and resins
    c. catalysts and initiators
    d. adhesives and catalysts _____

10. Initiators in polymer powder cause monomer molecules to permanently link together and form:
    a. short monomer chains
    c. long polymer forms
    b. long polymer chains
    d. short chain reactions
    _____

11. The initiator added to polymer powder is:
    a. hydrogen peroxide
    c. sodium hydroxide
    b. catalyst peroxide
    d. benzoyl peroxide
    _____

12. To ensure the proper curing when using nail enhancement products:
    a. use a variety of products
    b. intermix products as necessary
    c. mix manufacturer product lines
    d. do not mix manufacturer product lines
    _____

13. Acrylic (methacrylate) overlays and nail enhancements can be created using one color powder if the client wears:
    a. clear polish all the time
    c. semiliquid nail polish
    b. nail polish all the time
    d. natural colors all the time
    _____

14. The amount of monomer liquid and polymer powder used to create a bead is called the:
    a. dry bead
    c. powder ratio
    b. liquid bead
    d. mix ratio
    _____

15. If the consistency of a bead contains too little powder, the enhancement may not:
    a. file easily
    c. cure correctly
    b. balance easily
    d. polish easily
    _____

16. Surface moisture and oil on the natural nail plate can be removed with nail antiseptic or:
    a. nail dehydrators
    c. heavy primers
    b. corrosive agents
    d. nail hydrators
    _____

17. The use of acid-based nail primers may result in:
    a. skin burns or injury
    c. skin rejuvenation
    b. lifting of skin
    d. better adhesion
    _____

18. Acrylic (methacrylate) nail enhancements reach their ultimate strength in:
    a. 24 to 48 hours
    c. 30 to 45 minutes
    b. 5 to 10 hours
    d. 12 to 15 hours
    _____

19. Nail adhesives used to secure nail tips to natural nails are all based on:
    a. catalyst monomers
    c. acetone inhibitors
    b. cyanoacrylate polymers
    d. cyanoacrylate monomers
    _____

20. To prevent product contamination, a dappen dish should have:
    a. a loosely fitted lid
    b. a tightly fitted lid
    c. a large opening
    d. an evaporation lid _____

21. The shelf life of nail adhesives can be as short as:
    a. 1 year
    b. 8 months
    c. 6 months
    d. 2 years _____

22. Unused monomer poured back into the original container will cause product:
    a. spilling
    b. sensitivity
    c. customizing
    d. contamination _____

23. The type of glove recommended for nail salon services is:
    a. nylon polymer
    b. hard plastic
    c. latex polymer
    d. nitrile polymer _____

24. The area that should not be cut when applying multiuse nail forms is the:
    a. nail fold
    b. hyponychium
    c. cuticle fold
    d. nail root _____

25. The bead of product for shaping the free edge should have a:
    a. wet consistency
    b. balanced consistency
    c. medium consistency
    d. large consistency _____

26. The time required for a product to properly clean brushes is determined by:
    a. the technician
    b. the client
    c. the manufacturer's directions
    d. necessity _____

27. When placing the second ball of acrylic on the free edge, use a medium consistency and place on the nail plate below the first bead and:
    a. next to the side wall edge line and on the right side of the nail
    b. next to the free edge line within 1/8 inch of the nail
    c. next to the free edge line in the center of the nail
    d. on the nail plate within 1/8 inch of the cuticle area _____

28. For natural looking nails, the product application must be smooth and thin at the:
    a. eponychium, free edge, and base
    b. free edge and side walls
    c. side walls, free edge, and eponychium
    d. side walls, base, and free edge _____

29. In rebalancing acrylic (methacrylate) nail enhancements, the nail is thinned down and reduced in thickness and:
    a. the nail will be reduced in width
    b. the apex of the nail will be removed
    c. the nail will be filed
    d. the nail will be refinished   ____

30. The area between the existing acrylic product and new growth of the nail plate is the:
    a. thinned area   c. nail unit
    b. balance area   d. ledge   ____

CHAPTER 29—UV GELS

1. The ingredients used in UV gels are from a subfamily of acrylics called:
   a. monomers
   b. acrylates
   c. enhancements
   d. polymers ____

2. Recently developed UV gel technologies utilize chemistry from:
   a. monoacrylics
   b. polyacrylates
   c. methacrylates
   d. monomer powders ____

3. A short chain of monomers not long enough to be considered a polymer is a(n):
   a. additive
   b. adhesive
   c. oligomer
   d. resin ____

4. Newer UV gel systems use chemicals called:
   a. monomers
   b. urethane methacrylates
   c. adhesive based
   d. resin based ____

5. An advantage of UV gel systems is:
   a. color
   b. durability
   c. liquid polymer
   d. low odor ____

6. The UV gel application process differs from other types of nail enhancements; with a UV gel procedure:
   a. each layer of product is a different color when exposed to UV light
   b. each layer of product must cure or harden with exposure to UV light
   c. product is applied without the use of any UV light
   d. product must dry between layers with white lights ____

7. UV gel products are usually packaged in opaque pots or:
   a. dark bottles
   b. individual applications
   c. large tubes
   d. squeeze tubes ____

8. A measure of how much electricity a bulb consumes is:
   a. voltage
   b. amps
   c. wattage
   d. power ____

9. Brushes used in the application of UV gels are:
   a. human
   b. synthetic
   c. sable
   d. long ____

10. To improve the shelf life of nail adhesives, store them at room temperature between:
    a. 20°F and 40°F
    b. 45°F and 55°F
    c. 60°F and 85°F
    d. 90°F and 100°F ____

11. Nail tips applied with a UV gel procedure should be shortened and filed prior to the gel application to prevent:
    a. the client from spending extra time in the salon
    b. the gel seal from being broken during the filing procedure
    c. the gel application from curing correctly during the filing procedure
    d. skin irritations
    _____

12. The time required to cure each layer of a UV gel product is determined by:
    a. manufacturer's instructions   c. the client
    b. the length of the nail   d. the number of coats applied
    _____

13. UV gels cure with a tacky surface called a(n):
    a. second layer   c. inhibition layer
    b. contour layer   d. primary layer
    _____

14. The final layer of UV gel should be brushed under the free edge of the natural nail enhancement to create a(n):
    a. ledge   c. angle
    b. seal   d. adhesion
    _____

15. First UV gel is called the:
    a. base coat gel   c. sealing gel
    b. finishing gel   d. building gel
    _____

16. To reduce client skin irritation and sensitivity when applying the base coat gel:
    a. pull the UV gel quickly across the nail plate
    b. leave a tiny free margin between the UV gel and the skin
    c. remove the inhibition layer
    d. press hard with the brush
    _____

17. The oily shine on natural nails should be removed using:
    a. round circles   c. round strokes
    b. vertical strokes   d. firm pressure
    _____

18. UV gel enhancements must be rebalanced every:
    a. 2 to 3 weeks   c. 5 to 6 weeks
    b. 4 to 5 weeks   d. 6 to 8 weeks
    _____

19. The abrasive used to check and refine the nail contour for UV gel nails is:
    a. nonabrasive   c. medium abrasive
    b. fine abrasive   d. harsh abrasive
    _____

20. Third UV gel is called the finisher or:
    a. builder gel   c. building gel
    b. sealer gel   d. adhesion gel
    _____

CHAPTER 30—SEEKING EMPLOYMENT

1. Most professionals have become successful through self-motivation, energy, and:
   a. technical skills
   b. persistence
   c. talent
   d. opportunity _____

2. Of all the factors that affect licensing test performance, the most important is mastery of:
   a. technical skills
   b. organizing handouts
   c. course content
   d. school notes _____

3. When taking a licensure test, even if you have truly learned the material, it is still very beneficial to have:
   a. a well-organized notebook
   b. a detailed vocabulary list
   c. listening skills
   d. strong test-taking skills _____

4. The process of reaching logical conclusions by employing logical reasoning is:
   a. studying the night before the exam
   b. cramming the night before the exam
   c. marking skipped questions
   d. deductive reasoning _____

5. When reaffirming a goal by reviewing a number of important questions, it is recommended to perform a(n):
   a. personal inventory of characteristics and skills
   b. complete inventory of practical skills
   c. inventory of personal likes and qualities
   d. personal inventory of knowledge and skills _____

6. A salon owned by an individual or two or more partners with 3 to 40 styling stations is classified as a:
   a. full-service salon
   b. small independent salon
   c. independent salon chain
   d. neighborhood salon _____

7. Independent salon chains are basic or full-service salons and day spas consisting of five or more salons that are owned by:
   a. five or more partners
   b. large corporations
   c. one individual
   d. one individual or two or more partners _____

8. A form of chain salons that share a national name, consistent image, and business formula throughout are:
   a. franchise salons
   b. large chains
   c. privately owned
   d. business salons _____

9. A salon business that offers higher-priced services with luxurious extras is a:
   a. budget salon or day spa
   b. booth rental establishment
   c. basic value-priced operation
   d. high-end image salon or day spa ____

10. A written summary provided to employers of your education and work experience is a:
    a. job application
    b. résumé
    c. cover letter
    d. personal inventory ____

11. Skills mastered at other jobs that can be put to use in another position are called:
    a. transferable skills
    b. accomplishment skills
    c. salary references
    d. training skills ____

12. A bound collection of photos and documents used to showcase your skills and accomplishments is a(n):
    a. portfolio
    b. assessment
    c. resume
    d. summary ____

13. A technique of making contact with salons and professionals is called:
    a. gathering
    b. establishing
    c. advertising
    d. networking ____

14. After doing a salon site visit, it is important to send the salon representative a:
    a. résumé
    b. cover letter
    c. thank-you note
    d. declining note ____

15. When selecting and interviewing salons for potential employment opportunities, it is important that the stylist make:
    a. informed comparisons
    b. hasty choices
    c. no comparisons
    d. inappropriate remarks ____

16. After observing and targeting salons for employment opportunities, the next step would be to contact the establishments by:
    a. visiting the salon when they are busy
    b. sending a résumé and cover letter
    c. contacting the salon manger by phone
    d. completing a job application ____

17. When preparing for an interview, necessary employment information and materials include:
    a. identification and social security number
    b. drivers license and high school diploma
    c. social security number and cell phone number
    d. contact numbers and school certificate of completion _____

18. Issues and questions that cannot be included in an employment application or interview include:
    a. date of birth if applicant is younger than 18
    b. race, religion, date of birth, and national origin
    c. medical conditions and salary
    d. citizenship, drugs, and smoking _____

19. When you take pride in your work and commit yourself to doing a good job for your clients and employer, you have a strong:
    a. work ethic   c. employment advantage
    b. position statement   d. technical skill _____

20. On the day of a salon interview, a warm, friendly smile and confident posture will project a(n):
    a. good interview   c. false impression
    b. achievement   d. positive first impression _____

CHAPTER 31—ON THE JOB

1. Compared to cosmetology school, you will find that your real-world work schedule will be:
    a. more flexible   c. equally flexible
    b. less flexible   d. not at all flexible   ____

2. When seeking employment, it is important to be honest with yourself as you evaluate your skills to determine:
    a. how great your skills are
    b. the many services you are proficient at performing
    c. the type of position that is right for you
    d. the money that you can charge   ____

3. The number one thing to remember in a service business is that your work revolves around:
    a. serving your clients   c. the time of day
    b. how well you feel   d. how many hours you work   ____

4. To be a good team player requires that you practice and perfect your:
    a. telephone skills   c. people skills
    b. personal life   d. scheduled shifts   ____

5. The document that outlines all the duties and responsibilities of a particular position is a:
    a. duty list   c. daily chores summary
    b. job description   d. job document   ____

6. When you accept a job offer, what you actually get paid for your work is called:
    a. check   c. incentives
    b. cash   d. compensation   ____

7. In most salons the three standard methods of employee compensation are:
    a. salary, commission, and retail sales
    b. commission, salary plus commission, and employee incentives
    c. salary, commission, and salary plus commission
    d. check, commission, salary, and bonuses   ____

8. An excellent job opportunity for a new cosmetology school graduate is as a(n):
    a. assistant   c. practitioner
    b. platform artist   d. receptionist   ____

9. For the beginning salon professional without a clientele, the best compensation method would be:
   a. weekly
   b. commission only
   c. with no taxes
   d. a salary
   _____

10. Compensation paid to an employee as a direct result of the total amount of service dollars generated for the salon is:
    a. commission
    b. gratuities
    c. clientele
    d. salary
    _____

11. A compensation structure that is used to motivate and increase practitioner productivity is:
    a. tax-free salaries
    b. salary plus commission
    c. commission only
    d. regular compensation
    _____

12. Income provided in acknowledgment of satisfactory service that must be reported on one's income tax return is:
    a. tips
    b. taxes
    c. retail sales
    d. referrals
    _____

13. Employer and coworker feedback on technical abilities, career direction, and growth should be provided during a(n):
    a. client service
    b. referral program
    c. employee evaluation
    d. employee lunch break
    _____

14. To manage expenses and debts, financial planning includes a:
    a. mathematical genius
    b. personal budget
    c. personal diary
    d. free spending log
    _____

15. The practice of recommending and selling additional professional services to clients is:
    a. retail sales
    b. upselling services
    c. part of the duties and responsibilities
    d. part of the job description
    _____

16. Recommending and selling professional products to clients for at-home care is:
    a. economics
    b. commission
    c. advertising
    d. retailing
    _____

17. To be successful in sales, the practitioner must be ambitious and determined and have:
    a. a good client
    b. an assertive personality
    c. a good personality
    d. a personal preference
    _____

140

18. In the psychology of selling, it is the job of the practitioner to figure out the reason a person may want to buy a product and determine the client's:
    a. intelligence
    b. motives for buying salon products
    c. financial situation
    d. stress level
    ____

19. Clients whom you service on a regular basis are referred to as your:
    a. reliable clients
    b. good clients
    c. complaining clients
    d. client base
    ____

20. The process of scheduling clients for return visits to the salon is referred to as:
    a. selling
    b. suggestions
    c. rebooking
    d. referrals
    ____

CHAPTER 32—THE SALON BUSINESS

1. Being a successful businessperson requires experience, a genuine love of people, and solid:
   a. technical skills
   b. management skills
   c. business licenses
   d. insurance policies _____

2. Where allowed by state law, a desirable alternative salon ownership is the practice of:
   a. booth rental
   b. booth sales
   c. leased space
   d. unlicensed activity _____

3. When opening a salon, two of the most important factors in predicting the success of the business are:
   a. location and services
   b. visibility and products
   c. visibility and accessibility
   d. competition and products _____

4. When obtaining financing to open a business, it is essential to develop a(n):
   a. employee handbook
   b. business plan
   c. tax shelter
   d. service menu _____

5. The professional trained in the gathering of accurate financial information needed in developing a business plan is a(n):
   a. relative
   b. coworker
   c. vendor
   d. accountant _____

6. Purchasing the insurance required for operating a salon is the responsibility of the:
   a. salon owner
   b. building owner
   c. salon employee
   d. salon supplier _____

7. Another name for an individual owner with complete control of a business is:
   a. leader
   b. manager
   c. sole proprietor
   d. receptionist _____

8. In a partnership, two or more people share ownership, although the ownership shares may not always be:
   a. fair
   b. friendly
   c. equal
   d. operational _____

9. Incorporating is one of the best ways for a business owner to protect:
   a. personal assets
   b. unmanageable debts
   c. personal secrets
   d. supply inventory _____

10. A business advantage of a corporation when raising capital (money) is that a corporation may issue shares or:
   a. tax shelters
   b. stock certificates
   c. liability insurance
   d. business charters
   _____

11. To avoid any misunderstandings between contracting parties in the purchase a salon, the details of the sale should be written in the:
   a. building lease agreement
   b. business plan
   c. purchase and sales agreement
   d. professional name
   _____

12. Business records that are used to record all income are classified as:
   a. receipts
   b. invoices
   c. expenses
   d. retail
   _____

13. Records that help maintain an overstocking or shortage of supplies and are used to establish the net worth of a business are:
   a. invoice and revenue records
   b. purchase and inventory records
   c. sales and employee records
   d. expense and payroll records
   _____

14. Supplies used in the daily business operation are considered:
   a. retail supplies
   b. consumer supplies
   c. consumption supplies
   d. inventory supplies
   _____

15. Supplies purchased by a salon with the intention of selling these products to clients are:
   a. retail supplies
   b. consumption supplies
   c. special supplies
   d. client supplies
   _____

16. When planning and constructing the best physical layout for a salon, the primary concern should be:
   a. color scheme
   b. salon furniture
   c. salon carpeting
   d. maximum efficiency
   _____

17. To employees, a top priority for salon owners should be to always meet:
   a. employee evaluations
   b. incentives
   c. payroll obligations
   d. preferences
   _____

18. One of the most important duties of the receptionist is:
   a. booking appointments
   b. making reservations
   c. personal calls
   d. filing
   _____

19. The best form of advertising for a salon is a(n):
    a. radio spot   c. unhappy client
    b. newspaper   d. satisfied client   _____

20. An important aspect of a salon's financial success revolves around the sale of:
    a. gift certificates   c. key chains
    b. additional salon services   d. direct mail   _____

Part II: Answers to Exam Review for Cosmetology

CHAPTER 1—HISTORY AND CAREER OPPORTUNITIES

1. b	6. a	11. a
2. d	7. c	12. c
3. b	8. b	13. a
4. c	9. a	14. c
5. d	10. b	15. c

CHAPTER 2—LIFE SKILLS

1. b	6. c
2. c	7. c
3. a	8. a
4. c	9. d
5. b	10. a

CHAPTER 3—YOUR PROFESSIONAL IMAGE

1. d	6. b
2. a	7. a
3. d	8. a
4. a	9. a
5. d	10. c

CHAPTER 4—COMMUNICATING FOR SUCCESS

1. d	6. b	11. c
2. b	7. a	12. a
3. a	8. b	13. b
4. d	9. b	14. b
5. a	10. a	15. a

CHAPTER 5—INFECTION CONTROL: PRINCIPLES AND PRACTICES

1. c	11. d	21. a	31. a	41. a
2. b	12. a	22. b	32. b	42. b
3. a	13. c	23. c	33. a	43. c
4. b	14. a	24. b	34. d	44. a
5. b	15. a	25. d	35. a	45. a
6. d	16. b	26. a	36. b	46. a
7. c	17. a	27. b	37. c	47. a
8. c	18. b	28. c	38. a	48. b
9. d	19. c	29. d	39. b	49. a
10. a	20. a	30. c	40. d	50. c

CHAPTER 5—INFECTION CONTROL: PRINCIPLES AND PRACTICES (continued)

51. a	56. a	61. a	66. c	71. d
52. b	57. d	62. d	67. c	72. b
53. c	58. b	63. a	68. a	73. a
54. a	59. a	64. a	69. b	74. b
55. d	60. c	65. b	70. c	75. a

CHAPTER 6—GENERAL ANATOMY AND PHYSIOLOGY

1. a	15. b	29. a	43. d	57. b
2. b	16. b	30. c	44. a	58. c
3. a	17. c	31. d	45. d	59. a
4. d	18. c	32. b	46. b	60. c
5. c	19. b	33. a	47. a	61. b
6. b	20. c	34. c	48. d	62. c
7. c	21. a	35. c	49. b	63. b
8. a	22. d	36. b	50. d	64. c
9. a	23. b	37. a	51. b	65. b
10. d	24. a	38. d	52. b	66. a
11. b	25. b	39. a	53. b	
12. a	26. b	40. b	54. b	
13. c	27. c	41. c	55. c	
14. d	28. d	42. a	56. b	

CHAPTER 7—SKIN STRUCTURE AND GROWTH

1. b	8. a	15. b	22. d	29. d
2. c	9. c	16. c	23. a	30. a
3. b	10. a	17. d	24. c	31. c
4. a	11. b	18. a	25. b	32. b
5. c	12. a	19. c	26. c	33. a
6. d	13. b	20. b	27. d	34. b
7. b	14. a	21. a	28. a	35. d

CHAPTER 8—NAIL STRUCTURE AND GROWTH

1. b	6. a	11. c	16. a	21. d
2. c	7. c	12. a	17. a	22. c
3. b	8. a	13. d	18. b	23. b
4. d	9. b	14. a	19. d	24. a
5. d	10. b	15. c	20. a	25. d

CHAPTER 9—PROPERTIES OF THE HAIR AND SCALP

1. b	5. a	9. c	13. c	17. b
2. c	6. c	10. b	14. a	18. b
3. b	7. b	11. c	15. b	19. b
4. d	8. a	12. c	16. c	20. c

CHAPTER 9—PROPERTIES OF THE HAIR AND SCALP
(*continued*)

21. d	31. b	41. b	51. a	61. c
22. b	32. d	42. c	52. c	62. a
23. c	33. a	43. a	53. d	63. a
24. a	34. a	44. a	54. b	64. b
25. a	35. c	45. c	55. a	65. c
26. d	36. d	46. b	56. b	66. a
27. c	37. a	47. a	57. c	67. a
28. a	38. c	48. b	58. a	68. a
29. d	39. a	49. d	59. d	69. a
30. a	40. a	50. c	60. a	70. b

CHAPTER 10—BASICS OF CHEMISTRY

1. b	8. a	15. a	22. a	29. d
2. c	9. b	16. b	23. b	30. d
3. a	10. b	17. a	24. b	31. b
4. b	11. d	18. c	25. c	32. b
5. c	12. a	19. b	26. a	33. c
6. b	13. c	20. d	27. c	34. a
7. d	14. b	21. c	28. b	35. a

CHAPTER 11—BASICS OF ELECTRICITY

1. a	6. a	11. a	16. d	21. a
2. b	7. b	12. b	17. b	22. a
3. b	8. b	13. a	18. a	23. a
4. a	9. d	14. c	19. c	24. a
5. d	10. c	15. a	20. c	25. a

CHAPTER 12—PRINCIPLES OF HAIR DESIGN

1. b	7. d	13. b	19. b	25. a
2. a	8. a	14. d	20. a	26. d
3. c	9. b	15. a	21. d	27. c
4. a	10. a	16. a	22. a	28. d
5. c	11. d	17. c	23. c	29. a
6. d	12. a	18. a	24. a	30. b

CHAPTER 13—SHAMPOOING, RINSING, AND CONDITIONING

1. a	8. a	15. a	22. c	29. c
2. c	9. c	16. c	23. c	30. a
3. b	10. a	17. a	24. b	31. b
4. c	11. d	18. d	25. b	32. c
5. d	12. b	19. a	26. d	33. a
6. b	13. b	20. b	27. a	34. d
7. c	14. d	21. a	28. a	35. b

CHAPTER 14—HAIRCUTTING

1. b	14. a	27. c	40. c	53. c
2. c	15. d	28. d	41. a	54. d
3. b	16. b	29. b	42. b	55. b
4. d	17. c	30. b	43. d	56. a
5. a	18. c	31. c	44. b	57. b
6. b	19. c	32. a	45. a	58. c
7. c	20. d	33. b	46. c	59. a
8. d	21. a	34. c	47. c	60. b
9. a	22. b	35. a	48. b	61. c
10. d	23. d	36. b	49. b	62. b
11. b	24. b	37. b	50. c	63. a
12. b	25. b	38. d	51. c	64. d
13. c	26. b	39. b	52. b	65. a

CHAPTER 15—HAIRSTYLING

1. b	12. c	23. b	34. c	45. a
2. c	13. b	24. a	35. c	46. a
3. b	14. a	25. d	36. b	47. a
4. c	15. d	26. a	37. c	48. b
5. b	16. a	27. b	38. b	49. a
6. d	17. c	28. b	39. b	50. b
7. a	18. b	29. c	40. a	51. a
8. b	19. a	30. a	41. a	52. a
9. d	20. b	31. d	42. c	53. b
10. a	21. c	32. b	43. d	54. a
11. a	22. d	33. a	44. a	55. d

CHAPTER 16—BRAIDING AND BRAID EXTENSIONS

1. b	7. d	13. a	19. a	25. d
2. b	8. b	14. a	20. c	26. a
3. a	9. d	15. d	21. b	27. d
4. d	10. b	16. b	22. a	28. d
5. c	11. a	17. a	23. b	29. b
6. b	12. a	18. b	24. b	30. a

CHAPTER 17—WIGS AND HAIR ENHANCEMENTS

1. b	7. b	13. d	19. c	25. a
2. b	8. d	14. b	20. d	26. d
3. c	9. b	15. a	21. a	27. a
4. a	10. a	16. b	22. b	28. d
5. c	11. c	17. b	23. a	29. c
6. d	12. c	18. d	24. d	30. a

CHAPTER 18—CHEMICAL TEXTURE SERVICES

1. b	14. b	27. a	40. a	53. d
2. d	15. d	28. b	41. a	54. b
3. a	16. a	29. b	42. b	55. b
4. b	17. b	30. a	43. d	56. c
5. a	18. c	31. d	44. b	57. a
6. b	19. d	32. b	45. a	58. a
7. b	20. a	33. c	46. b	59. c
8. d	21. b	34. b	47. a	60. b
9. b	22. a	35. a	48. c	61. c
10. a	23. d	36. b	49. b	62. b
11. c	24. a	37. d	50. b	63. c
12. b	25. b	38. c	51. b	64. d
13. a	26. c	39. a	52. b	65. c

CHAPTER 19—HAIRCOLORING

1. b	15. b	29. c	43. c	57. b
2. a	16. b	30. b	44. b	58. a
3. d	17. d	31. d	45. d	59. b
4. a	18. b	32. c	46. c	60. b
5. a	19. b	33. a	47. c	61. d
6. c	20. d	34. c	48. c	62. b
7. a	21. a	35. b	49. b	64. d
8. b	22. b	36. d	50. d	65. b
9. c	23. c	37. b	51. b	65. d
10. d	24. d	38. a	52. d	66. d
11. a	25. c	39. c	53. a	67. b
12. b	26. d	40. b	54. c	68. d
13. d	27. a	41. b	55. b	69. b
14. b	28. b	42. a	56. c	70. c

CHAPTER 20—SKIN DISEASES AND DISORDERS

1. b	7. d	13. a	19. d	25. d
2. d	8. d	14. b	20. b	26. c
3. a	9. b	15. c	21. a	27. b
4. b	10. d	16. b	22. c	28. d
5. c	11. a	17. b	23. b	29. b
6. b	12. d	18. a	24. a	30. a

CHAPTER 21—HAIR REMOVAL

1. b	6. a	11. a	16. d	21. d
2. c	7. a	12. d	17. a	22. b
3. a	8. b	13. d	18. b	23. a
4. d	9. b	14. c	19. c	24. a
5. b	10. d	15. b	20. b	25. b

CHAPTER 22—FACIALS

1. b	11. b	21. b	31. b	41. b
2. d	12. b	22. a	32. d	42. c
3. c	13. d	23. d	33. c	43. b
4. a	14. a	24. c	34. b	44. d
5. b	15. d	25. a	35. a	45. a
6. c	16. c	26. b	36. c	46. c
7. a	17. c	27. a	37. d	47. b
8. d	18. b	28. b	38. a	48. a
9. b	19. b	29. d	39. b	49. d
10. c	20. a	30. c	40. c	50. c

CHAPTER 23—FACIAL MAKEUP

1. c	7. c	13. c	19. a	25. c
2. d	8. b	14. b	20. b	26. a
3. a	9. a	15. c	21. b	27. c
4. a	10. c	16. d	22. b	28. b
5. b	11. d	17. c	23. d	29. b
6. b	12. b	18. a	24. a	30. b

CHAPTER 24—NAIL DISEASES AND DISORDERS

1. a	6. d	11. c	16. a
2. a	7. c	12. c	17. a
3. b	8. d	13. a	18. b
4. c	9. a	14. b	19. a
5. b	10. a	15. a	20. b

CHAPTER 25—MANICURING

1. b	8. c	15. d	22. d	29. c
2. c	9. b	16. a	23. a	30. b
3. b	10. d	17. a	24. c	31. a
4. d	11. c	18. c	25. b	32. a
5. b	12. c	19. b	26. c	33. d
6. b	13. b	20. c	27. a	34. a
7. a	14. b	21. d	28. b	35. c

CHAPTER 26—PEDICURING

1. b	6. a	11. b	16. d	21. a
2. c	7. d	12. a	17. a	22. b
3. b	8. b	13. b	18. d	23. c
4. d	9. c	14. c	19. c	24. b
5. c	10. b	15. b	20. b	25. d

CHAPTER 27—NAIL TIPS, WRAPS, AND NO-LIGHT GELS

1. b	6. a	11. d	16. b
2. a	7. b	12. c	17. d
3. d	8. d	13. d	18. d
4. b	9. c	14. b	19. d
5. c	10. a	15. c	20. b

CHAPTER 28—ACRYLIC (METHACRYLATE) NAILS

1. b	7. b	13. b	19. d	25. c
2. d	8. a	14. d	20. b	26. c
3. a	9. c	15. c	21. c	27. c
4. d	10. b	16. a	22. d	28. c
5. b	11. d	17. a	23. d	29. b
6. c	12. d	18. a	24. b	30. d

CHAPTER 29—UV GELS

1. b	6. b	11. b	16. b
2. c	7. d	12. a	17. b
3. c	8. c	13. c	18. a
4. b	9. b	14. b	19. c
5. d	10. c	15. a	20. b

CHAPTER 30—SEEKING EMPLOYMENT

1. b	6. b	11. a	16. b
2. c	7. d	12. a	17. a
3. d	8. a	13. d	18. b
4. d	9. d	14. c	19. a
5. a	10. b	15. a	20. d

CHAPTER 31—ON THE JOB

1. b	6. d	11. b	16. d
2. c	7. c	12. a	17. c
3. a	8. a	13. c	18. b
4. c	9. d	14. b	19. d
5. b	10. a	15. b	20. c

CHAPTER 32—THE SALON BUSINESS

1. b	6. a	11. c	16. d
2. a	7. c	12. a	17. c
3. c	8. c	13. b	18. a
4. b	9. a	14. c	19. d
5. d	10. b	15. a	20. b

NOTES